Gut Health for Life

Eat to Live Pain Free

Table of Contents

MY STORY 1

INTRODUCTION 9

CHAPTER 1: THE INFLAMMATION EQUATION 11

CHAPTER 2: QUENCHING FLAMES—FOODS THAT COOL
DOWN INFLAMMATION 27

CHAPTER 3: CRAFTING AN ANTI-INFLAMMATORY
BLUEPRINT 41

CHAPTER 4: DAWN DELIGHTS—A GUIDE TO
ANTI-INFLAMMATORY BREAKFASTS 59

CHAPTER 5: MIDDAY MORSELS—NOURISHING THE NOON 75

CHAPTER 6: EVENING ELIXIRS—NURTURING THE NIGHT.................89

CHAPTER 7: TWILIGHT TEMPTATIONS—OFFERING
SNACKS WITH ANTI-INFLAMMATORY INTENT 101

CHAPTER 8: WEAVING WELLNESS INTO LIFE'S FABRIC.................115

CONCLUSION...129

REFERENCES...131

My Story

I get it, you've tried every approach to improving your health and well-being. You may have even experienced some improvement in your gut health and maybe even some weight loss, but it always comes back—sometimes with reinforcements. You may feel like a failure—like you're constantly depriving yourself only to end up right back where you started.

There is a way to escape this all-too-familiar pattern once and for all. There is a blueprint for real, lasting improvements that doesn't require unsustainable restrictions or unhealthy obsessions. If you give me the opportunity, I will shatter the myths of quick-fix approaches and teach you how to develop a positive, holistic lifestyle that puts you firmly in control of your health.

I'm here to tell you that if I can do it, so can you. I want to share my personal story with you as a way to illustrate that anyone has the ability to cultivate a new lifestyle and change their future.

Time for a Change

Every personal transformation story begins when the right motivations strike you at the right time. My experience was no different. Like any other middle-aged person who is overweight, my health began to suffer. Not only was I prediabetic, but doctors had also diagnosed me with high blood pressure. When I think about this period of time, I describe it as living in a body that was working against me. I would wake up in the morning and everything would ache. Even simple tasks like walking up stairs would be tiring. I thought, *I am too young to feel this old*. I remember feeling drained and physically uncomfortable.

I knew things needed to change, but the spark to finally take action never seemed to ignite. Unfortunately, the discomfort and doctors' pleas were not enough to motivate me to push past my fear of failure and make significant changes.

Wake-Up Call

In the midst of these challenging emotions, I got a literal wake-up call. My father, who is diabetic, phoned me from 1,000 miles away. He found himself on the ground, unable to recall how he had gotten there, and in need of help. He couldn't move or get up on his own. I felt helpless as I tried to coordinate care for him from a distance.

That day, I learned that 911 isn't a universal national service. One must call the local police or emergency line for that specific location, and of course, I didn't know any of that. In the world of cell phones, who knows the area code for someone 1,000 miles away! The five minutes it took me to find and get ahold of emergency services in his area felt like an hour to me. At any moment, I feared things could get worse.

Eventually, an ambulance arrived and took him to the hospital. His kidneys had failed, and the time had come for him to be placed on dialysis. The thought of what might have happened if he were unable to reach me was chilling. He lived alone, and while we knew his kidneys were getting worse, we did not anticipate this immediate of a crisis.

I visited with him in the hospital, accompanied by his sister, my Aunt Helen. Seeing someone we admired and trusted struggling with the consequences of lifestyle choices was devastating. Our deep conversations during these visits impacted me greatly.

He wasn't the only one having an impact on me. There were other sick people of advanced age in the hospital with him. I could feel their pain as I saw them fight for their very lives.

I wondered, H*ad these people lived like me? Did they have productive and full lives? Did they have hopes and dreams at their age that they now must set aside in* *favor of just surviving?* The future I was being shown to me was not how I pictured my life ending up.

It was during one of my deep conversations with my Aunt Helen that I realized these things were impacting her too. We spoke about how we must take care of ourselves because this body is all we have. It really hit me in that moment. That conversation was a turning point for me.

I still had doubts and fear. There was the resistance to changing a lifestyle I had been used to for so long. Eventually, though, the insecurity and doubt I had about my future outweighed the desire to keep things the same.

So, there I was, at my lowest point physically and mentally. Your current feelings may be similar: fearful of change, fearful of failure, but also fearful of the future shaped by poor habits.

Time for a Change

At this point, even the internet had figured out that I was looking for a way out of my current lifestyle. I knew there was false information out there, and my fear used that as a crutch to stop me from taking action. The visit with the doctor was surprisingly routine. They examined my BMI, posed a few questions, confirmed my A1C levels were diabetic, and the high blood pressure was still elevated. I knew I couldn't live like this, and it was time for a change.

There was an upcoming special event for my son in August. Knowing that I was accountable to this date to improve my health and well-being filled me with the motivation to set a great example for my son and to be able to fully enjoy the celebration. Resolute and determined, I set out to make it happen. I truly believe success only happens when you know the importance of your goals, so I wrote down my "why" and my "when" and read them back every day.

My activity subtly changed over time. I found myself taking longer walks with my wife and dog, and I played sports more frequently with my children. I wasn't eating to the point of discomfort anymore, so I felt well enough to be active.

I also got serious about eating healthy, both for weight loss and gut health. I focused on fruits, vegetables, small portions of lean meat, healthy grains, legumes, and nuts. This made a tremendous difference in my overall health and was not very hard to accomplish.

Eating to improve your well-being is important no matter how you approach your well-being. I'm not referring to going on a diet but, rather, adopting a holistic approach to eating that works with your body. This book was borne out of the changes I made through this process. It is not a diet (however I did lose significant weight). It is a lifestyle choice! An approach to well being that not only made me feel great, but it allowed me to enjoy my life again!

I began to exercise as well. I focused primarily on two objectives: 1) getting outside to enjoy walking, playing sports and having fun, and 2) Strength Training with weights!

Sure enough, my body went from simply losing fat to gaining muscle as a result, and that's when I saw the physical change. It was an amazing confidence boost, I felt more like myself, and I was proud of the progress I was seeing.

This period of my life marked when I learned so much about food and the role it plays in how we feel. I noticed that by changing my nutritional intake I didn't feel deprived; I felt fueled and invigorated. I could feel food working *with* my body, rather than against it. These intentional changes—which I was too fearful to take on at first—now felt as if they had been my habits all my life.

Food doesn't run the show anymore; I do. I am in control of my future and my choices. Knowing that makes me a better worker, husband, father, and friend. This journey hasn't just given me the potential to live longer but also the ability to have more impact on the world while I'm here.

There could be no greater prize than more time with my family because I feel better. A longer life with the people I cherish is more important to me than how I look in the mirror.

Food doesn't run the show anymore; I do. I am in control of my future and my choices. Knowing that makes me a better worker, husband, father, and friend. This journey hasn't just given me the potential to live longer but also the ability to have more impact on the world while I'm here.

Lessons From My Journey

Now, if all that was too much for you, and you just want the wisdom, here you go!

Write Down Your Why and When

The most vital part of your journey is knowing your motivation. Writing down your "why" and your "when"—a date by which you want to have reached a tangible goal—helps to solidify your commitment to this transformation.

For me, this written record of my motivation became a constant reminder that I would look at daily. So, seriously, take a break to ponder your own reasons and goals, and write them down now. You wouldn't be reading this book if you didn't have goals in mind, so take the time to streamline your motivations and create a written record of them. This book will still be here when you come back.

If you don't consolidate your "why" and your "when," it is significantly harder to understand the steps to take to reach your goals and to recognize and celebrate your progress along the way. This, in turn, makes it more difficult to remain diligent when motivation wanes.

Therefore, this is the single most important step of your journey. Consider sharing your "why" and "when" with your loved ones to both reaffirm your commitment and build an instant support network!

Maximize benefits With Hydration and Food Tracking

Drink plenty of water, over-hydrate, to imrove well being. Giving your body plenty of what it needs to flush things out is essential. Also, remember to take a prebiotic and probiotic to keep your digestion track moving.

Additionally, it's important to keep track of how certain foods affect how you feel. For me, eating certain foods were uncomfortable, and by eliminating them, I improved my well being

Strength Training Over Cardio

As you will be eating different foods that energize you in different way, you don't need cardio to burn extra calories, but you do need to build strength. Focus on walking at first if that's all you can do, then eventually work your way up to strength training for 30 minutes, three to four days a week. This is more than enough exercise to promote muscle growth.

Remember, This Is a Journey

As you progress, you will encounter setbacks. Track the long-term trends, not the short-term fluctuations, and don't get discouraged.

If you make a mistake, jump right back on the wagon. Don't let one bad meal or one bad day derail you completely.

There's always a path back to your journey, no matter how far you've strayed. The only way to fail at this is to give up before you meet your goal.

Now that you have learned about my journey it's time to get started on yours. We'll start at the beginning, explain how it all works, and soon, you'll be set on a path for the same remarkable success!

Introduction

In a world where chronic inflammation is silently but steadily becoming a widespread concern affecting millions of people with its insidious reach, the importance of addressing this health challenge cannot be overstressed. Mitigating its impacts is not just about managing discomfort; it's about fundamentally enhancing our quality of life. This book is born out of the recognition of an urgent need: to combat inflammation through the powerful tools of diet and lifestyle choices. The cornerstone of our discussion is the profound impact of anti-inflammatory foods and the transformative potential of making informed lifestyle adjustments.

At the heart of this guide lies a simple yet profound point of learning: The foods we eat and the way we live have the power to significantly increase or reduce the levels of inflammation within our bodies, thereby hugely impacting our overall health and well-being. Throughout the chapters ahead, we'll explore not just the science behind inflammation and its effects on the body but also practical and delicious ways to introduce anti-inflammatory foods into your daily meals.

This book is structured to offer you clarity and ease of navigation, firstly illuminating why gut health is so vital and then identifying the potential culprits behind inflammation and highlighting the unsung heroes of anti-inflammatory foods. I will also provide a curated selection of potential groceries to buy and meal ideas to try to simplify your shopping experience and ensure that you have the right ingredients on hand to try some anti-inflammatory breakfasts, lunches, and dinners. These ingredients transform these recipes into more than just meals; they are stepping stones toward a life of vitality and vigor.

If you are seeking not just to live but to thrive, this book is for you. Whether you're battling inflammation or aiming to prevent it, the guidance provided within these pages is invaluable. You hold in your hands the promise of improved well-being that extends beyond mere symptom management to the very essence of health.

As we embark on this journey together, I bring not only a deep-seated passion for holistic health but also a commitment to providing reliable, easily digestible information—much like the anti-inflammatory foods presented. My mission is to empower you with knowledge and practical tools that will enable you to make choices that foster a healthier, more vibrant life.

I invite you to engage actively with the content of this book. Let each page challenge you to rethink your relationship with food and lifestyle choices, and allow every recipe to inspire you to embrace the delicious possibilities of anti-inflammatory eating.

The path to an anti-inflammatory life is not just a possibility; it's a choice that begins with turning this page. So, let's begin this transformative journey together—one meal at a time—toward a future where vitality and well-being are within your grasp.

Chapter 1:

The Inflammation Equation

While we often only think about inflammation in its harmful, chronic form, in the short term, it is actually a testament to our bodies' inherent resilience—a biological alarm system designed to protect and heal us. It is when this system misfires or overstays its welcome that it morphs from protector to perpetrator, laying the groundwork for a myriad of chronic conditions. This chapter peels back the layers of this complex physiological process, shedding light on its dual nature, as well as its underlying mechanisms, manifestations, and long-term implications when unaddressed.

The Science Behind Inflammation: How It Affects Your Body

Inflammation is as old as human existence; it is the body's immediate response to injury or invasion by harmful entities. At its core, it is a protective response—the immune system's attempt to isolate affected areas, eliminate aggressors, and initiate tissue repair. However, when this transient defender turns into a chronic condition, it silently undermines our health and paves the way for diseases that insidiously compromise our well-being.

Inflammation's Dual Nature

In its short-term form, inflammation is a vivid demonstration of the body's defense mechanism. Picture a bustling city (your body) suddenly facing an unexpected disruption (injury or infection). The immediate response involves directing essential traffic (blood flow) to the affected area to bring in law enforcement and medical personnel (white blood cells and immune factors) who can manage the situation, clear debris, and facilitate recovery. This process is marked by well-known signs: redness, heat, swelling, pain, and loss of function, which are essentially the body's distress signals calling for attention and care.

However, when the cause of this disruption lingers or your body's regulatory mechanisms falter, this acute response doesn't recede. Instead, it transitions into a chronic state—akin to a city under siege— where the constant alert status begins to wear down its infrastructure and inhabitants. Chronic inflammation is a silent epidemic operating beneath the radar and contributing to the development and progression of many health conditions including heart disease, diabetes, cancer, and neurodegenerative issues.

Biological Mechanisms

To comprehend inflammation's impact, an understanding of its biological underpinnings is essential. At the molecular level, inflammation is triggered by physiological signals—cytokines and chemokines, which are proteins released by the impacted cells. These chemical signals recruit immune cells to the site of the injury or infection. The immune cells, in turn, release a plethora of substances that increase blood flow and cell wall permeability, therefore allowing more immune cells to reach and assist the problem area.

Under normal health circumstances, this process is tightly regulated by your body's natural reactions, ensuring that the inflammatory response is proportional to the issue at hand and resolved once the threat to your body is neutralized. However, with chronic inflammation, this regulation is disrupted. The signals persist, leading to the continuous recruitment of immune cells and the prolonged presence of inflammatory substances; this can eventually cause tissue damage and systemic effects.

Symptoms and Signs

Recognizing the manifestations of chronic inflammation is crucial for early intervention. Unlike its acute counterpart, chronic inflammation rarely announces itself with clear signals. Instead, it presents subtly with symptoms that can be easy to dismiss or misattribute: persistent fatigue, unexplained discomfort, digestive issues, or general malaise. More specific signs—such as joint pain, stiffness, or skin issues like eczema—may also point to underlying inflammatory issues. These symptoms are the body's subdued alarm bells signaling an imbalance that merits attention and action.

Long-Term Effects

The repercussions of prolonged inflammation reach far and wide, subsequently influencing nearly every organ in our bodies and contributing to a spectrum of diseases. For example, chronic inflammation plays a pivotal role in the development of atherosclerosis, wherein inflammatory processes contribute to plaque formation and resultant cardiovascular disease. Similarly, in the realm of metabolic health, insulin resistance and type-2 diabetes are closely linked to inflammation.

Moreover, our brains are not immune to these inflammatory effects. Neuro-inflammation is implicated in conditions ranging from depression to Alzheimer's disease, illustrating its broad impact on cognitive and emotional health.

In addressing inflammation, the goal is not to extinguish this essential biological response but to modulate its activity and ensure that it serves its protective role without veering into pathological territory. This nuanced approach involves lifestyle and dietary strategies aimed at calming the inflammatory response and, therefore, fostering an environment in which your body's natural healing processes can prevail.

By understanding the science behind inflammation and its profound impact on our bodies, we equip ourselves with the knowledge to make informed decisions about our health, thus paving the way for interventions that not only alleviate symptoms but also address the root causes of disease. The management and prevention of chronic inflammation are pivotal elements in any quest for lasting health and vitality, and this underscores the critical role of lifestyle choices in shaping our well-being.

Identifying Common Inflammatory Foods to Avoid

To mitigate the effects of chronic inflammation, we must take a careful look at our dietary landscape. Central to this endeavor is the identification and subsequent avoidance of foods that are catalysts for inflammatory responses. The usual suspects include refined sugars and saturated fats—common components of the modern diet that stealthily exacerbate our bodies' inflammatory processes. Refined sugars—found in copious amounts in soft drinks, pastries, and candies—instigate a rapid increase in blood sugar levels; this is a common trigger for a cascade of events that culminate in the release of pro-inflammatory messengers. Likewise, saturated fats—heavily present in red meats, dairy, and processed foods—follow a similar trajectory, consequently inciting the immune system into an unnecessary state of alert that perpetuates inflammation.

Beyond these overt antagonists lies a subtler, more insidious contributor to inflammation: food sensitivities. Unlike allergies—which declare themselves with immediate, sometimes life-threatening symptoms—sensitivities operate under the radar, quietly fueling inflammation with every unsuspecting bite. Gluten and dairy are common sources of dietary sensitivities that lead to a silent uproar within the digestive system and beyond. For some, the ingestion of gluten—a protein found in wheat, barley, and rye—initiates an inflammatory response that can ripple out and affect far more than just their gut. Likewise, dairy's presence can be protested by bodies that are unable to properly digest lactose or casein—a sugar and a protein found in milk, respectively.

Additionally, the role of processed foods in inflammation cannot be overstated. These dietary shortcuts are laden with additives and preservatives, offering convenience at the expense of health. Phosphates, for instance, are used to enhance flavor and moisture retention in meats, but they negatively impact your body's ability to utilize minerals like calcium and magnesium, leading to tighter muscles, reduced blood flow, and thus higher levels of inflammation. Similarly, nitrates—which are found in cured products— extend a product's shelf life, while potentially shortening ours by promoting inflammation. High sodium content is another hallmark of processed foods that further exacerbates the issue by contributing to hypertension and cardiovascular strain, both of which are intimately linked to inflammation.

Navigating this complex dietary terrain necessitates a keen eye for ingredient labels—a skill that, once honed, becomes an indispensable ally in the fight against inflammation. While the front of a package may boast health claims, the truth lies in the small print. Ingredients are listed by quantity from most to least present, and thus, they can offer insight into the product's composition. Components like "hydrogenated" or "partially hydrogenated" oils signal the presence of trans fats, which are notorious for their inflammatory potential. Additionally, high-fructose corn syrup—a type of refined sugar—lurks in many processed foods ranging from bread to salad dressings. Even products marketed as "healthy" can be deceptive with labels cloaked in terms that obscure the presence of inflammatory agents.

As a result, knowledge is power. Understanding the inflammatory potential of certain foods and ingredients equips us with the ability to make informed dietary choices. It allows us to sidestep the pitfalls of modern eating habits and steers our course toward a diet that supports rather than undermines our bodies' natural defenses against inflammation. Through vigilance and informed choices, we can recalibrate our diets, transforming our meals from sources of inflammation into vehicles of health and vitality.

The Anti-Inflammatory Food Pyramid: A Visual Guide

An anti-inflammatory food pyramid can illuminate the path to a diet that not only nourishes but also protects our bodies. This pyramid, unlike its more traditional counterpart, is reimagined and restructured by placing a vibrant array of fruits and vegetables, instead of grains, at its base—the cornerstone of anti-inflammatory eating. Fruits and vegetables are not merely food; they're a powerful source of phytonutrients, antioxidants, and fibers, each of which can contribute to your body's defense against inflammation. Variety is key; from the deep blues and purples of berries rich in anthocyanins to the bright oranges and yellows of citruses and squashes bursting with vitamin C and carotenoids, each color of fruit or veggies offers a different selection of nutrients.

Ascending the pyramid, the second tier introduces further pivotal anti-inflammatory soldiers: whole grains, lean proteins, and healthy fats. With their unrefined textures and intact nutrients, whole grains offer more than mere sustenance; they provide a steady source of energy that stabilizes blood sugar levels and curbs the inflammatory responses that are triggered by spikes and dips. Quinoa, brown rice, and oats are the bearers of B vitamins and minerals that can also contribute to your body's resilience against inflammation.

Lean proteins occupy an equally crucial space in this tier. Protein sources offer the physiological building blocks necessary for cell repair and growth, allowing us to heal and develop. Yet, your choice of protein matters: Fish—particularly oily fish like salmon and mackerel, which are rich in omega-3 fatty acids—offer anti-inflammatory benefits beyond mere protein content. Additionally, including poultry and legumes in your diet allows you to avoid the inflammatory saturated fats present in red and cured meats, providing alternatives that can satisfy both your body's needs and your palate's preferences.

Healthy fats round out this middle tier, challenging long-held misconceptions about the role of fats in health. The monounsaturated and polyunsaturated fats found in olive oil, avocados, and nuts do more than enrich our meals with flavor; they also weave a protective web against inflammation by stripping "bad" cholesterol from our artery walls and thus providing for smoother blood flow. Likewise, flaxseeds, chia seeds, and walnuts are not merely additions to our diet; they're integral components of an anti-inflammatory lifestyle. This serves as a testament to the power of fats when chosen wisely and consumed judiciously.

At the pinnacle of the pyramid reside those foods that, while not inherently inflammatory, are to be approached with mindfulness. This apex does not prohibit the intake of the foods listed within it but, rather, acts as a gentle reminder to prioritize balance and moderation. Alcohol and dark chocolate, when enjoyed in small quantities, weave pleasure into the fabric of our diets without tipping the scales toward inflammation, for instance. The pyramid's peak is where we find space for culinary indulgence tempered by the wisdom of restraint.

This anti-inflammatory food pyramid is a blueprint for eating that intertwines pleasure with health and taste with nourishment. It acknowledges the complexity of dietary choices in the modern world and offers a compass by which to navigate the vast sea of nutritional information. This is not only a tool but also a symbol of the power we hold over our health—a power we can exercise with every meal and bite.

In this reimagined food pyramid, layers interlock by supporting and enhancing each other. The base of fruits and vegetables provides the antioxidants and fibers necessary for combating inflammation, while the middle tiers supply the protein and fats essential for repair, growth, and protection. The tip, though modest in its contributions, offers a nod to the human need for the enjoyment of food without sacrificing health on the altar of pleasure.

So, this pyramid is more than a dietary model; it's a reflection of a holistic approach to eating and living—one that recognizes the interplay between food, body, and health. Transcending the restrictive simplicity of "eat this, not that," this guide invites us to develop a deeper understanding of how what we eat influences not just our physical well-being but also our overall quality of life. It challenges us to look beyond calories and nutrients to see food as a source of life, vitality, and healing.

In adopting this pyramid as our guide, we can explore the bounty that nature offers by experimenting with flavors, textures, and combinations that delight our senses while nurturing our bodies. This enables us to learn to listen to our bodies and discern what nourishes and what depletes—what heals and what harms. This journey is one of empowerment that offers us the tools to shape our health and our lives one meal at a time.

The Gut-Inflammation Connection: Why Gut Health Matters

The gut plays a leading role in our health (or lack thereof), orchestrating a complex interplay between our diet, microbiome, and levels of inflammation. The gut is often referred to as the body's "second brain," and it is home to a vast ecosystem of bacteria—trillions, in fact—that influence far more than just digestion. This microbial universe is teeming with life, and it exerts a profound impact on our bodies' inflammatory response, tipping the scales toward health or disease based on its composition and balance.

Gut Microbiome and Inflammation

The gut microbiome is bustling with microbial inhabitants that engage in a symbiotic relationship with their human host. These microscopic denizens perform crucial functions from fermenting dietary fiber and developing short-chain fatty acids—and thus improving nutrient absorption and energy regulation—to synthesizing essential vitamins. However, their influence extends beyond the confines of the gut, affecting your systemic inflammation levels and, by extension, your overall health.

A balanced gut microbiome allows beneficial bacteria to flourish, keeps pathogenic species in check, and enables the immune system to operate with precision. In contrast, dysbiosis—a state of microbial imbalance—upsets this delicate equilibrium: Harmful bacteria gain the upper hand, disrupt gut integrity, and allow inflammatory substances to escape into the bloodstream, which can ignite inflammatory responses throughout the body. Thus, the composition of your gut microbiome plays a huge part in modulating inflammation, and diet plays a central role in shaping this microbial landscape.

Leaky Gut Syndrome

Central to gut health and inflammation is the concept of intestinal permeability; when too high, this is colloquially known as *leaky gut syndrome*. Under normal conditions, the gut barrier is a selectively permeable vigilant gatekeeper that allows nutrients to pass into your bloodstream while barring harmful substances. However, certain factors including stress, toxins, and, critically, diet can compromise this barrier's function.

With a leaky gut, the tight junctions that seal the gut lining loosen, creating gaps through which bacteria, toxins, and undigested food particles can make their way into your bloodstream. This breach triggers an immune response, in turn causing an inflammatory reaction that can ripple throughout the body. The implications of this are far-reaching, linking leaky gut syndrome to a variety of inflammatory conditions ranging from autoimmune diseases to metabolic syndrome.

Probiotics and Prebiotics

Probiotics and prebiotics are invaluable allies in your battle to regulate your gut microbiome. Probiotics—live, beneficial bacteria—offer a direct means of enriching the gut's microbial population, thus fostering diversity and resilience. Found in fermented foods like yogurt, kefir, and sauerkraut, these microscopic benefactors colonize the gut, therefore reinforcing its barrier and competing with harmful bacteria for resources and space.

Prebiotics, on the other hand, are nourishment for these beneficial bacteria. Derived from dietary fibers found in foods such as garlic, onions, bananas, and asparagus, prebiotics fuel the growth and activity of probiotics, thereby enhancing their beneficial impacts on gut health and inflammation. Together, probiotics and prebiotics work to maintain gut integrity, support immune function, and modulate inflammation, illustrating the power of diet in influencing health.

Dietary Changes for Gut Health

Given the central role of diet in shaping the gut microbiome and, by extension, influencing inflammation, dietary adjustments are the most practical strategy for promoting gut health. A shift to a diet rich in whole foods—characterized by an abundance of fruits, vegetables, whole grains, and lean proteins—lays the groundwork for a healthy gut. Such a diet provides a diverse array of nutrients and fibers, fostering a balanced microbial ecosystem that is conducive to reduced inflammation.

Crucially, this dietary approach involves not just the inclusion of beneficial foods but also the minimization of foods that are detrimental to gut health. Processed foods high in sugar, unhealthy fats, and additives can contribute to dysbiosis and increased intestinal permeability. Similarly, excessive alcohol and caffeine intake can also disrupt your gut barrier, leading to or exacerbating leaky gut syndrome as a result.

In practical terms, implementing dietary changes for gut health involves a gradual transition toward a more plant-centric diet that will introduce pro- and prebiotics through fermented and high-fiber foods, respectively. Moreover, an awareness of food choices that can support or undermine gut integrity is needed.

Such understanding and mindful decision-making allows your diet to be more than a means of nourishment, also providing a tool for cultivating gut health, quelling inflammation, and by extension, fostering systemic well-being. Through conscious dietary choices, we can wield the power to influence our internal microbial universes and steer them toward balance and health. This interconnectedness of diet, microbiome, and well-being highlights the gut's pivotal role in the holistic health equation.

Decoding Food Labels: Hidden Inflammatory Ingredients

As we have previously touched on, modern food labels demand a discerning eye to pierce through the veil of marketing and uncover the truth of nutritional content. This is a vital step in identifying and avoiding hidden inflammatory agents that often lurk unnoticed in packaged foods. For instance, certain food additives have a proclivity to incite inflammatory responses, transforming seemingly innocuous foods into hidden harbingers of harm.

Preservatives are designed to extend shelf life, but they frequently double as instigators of inflammation. Sodium benzoate and potassium sorbate, in particular—while effective at inhibiting mold growth—have been implicated in activating inflammatory pathways within the body.

Similarly, artificial flavors and colors are added to enhance appeal, but they also often harbor their own inflammatory potential. Monosodium glutamate (MSG) is a flavor enhancer that is ubiquitous in processed foods, and it has been associated with headaches and other symptoms related to inflammation in sensitive individuals. Likewise, the artificial dyes that imbue foods with vibrant, eye-catching hues have not escaped scrutiny, with studies hinting at their role in exacerbating inflammatory conditions, particularly in children.

The task of deciphering food labels is further complicated by marketing strategies that adeptly mask the presence of these inflammatory agents. Terms like "natural flavors" and "spices" may seem benign, yet their ambiguity can hide a host of additives. Similarly, health claims adorning packaging—proclamations of "low fat," "reduced sugar," or "enriched with vitamins"—often distract from less desirable, hidden ingredients. This misdirection plays upon the consumer's desire for healthful choices, obfuscating the presence of additives that may undermine those very intentions.

The debate surrounding organic versus nonorganic foods adds another layer to the complexity of food choices and their impact on inflammation. Pesticides and herbicides—the chemicals commonly used on nonorganic crops—carry their own inflammatory risks. These substances are designed to kill pests and weeds, but they can also disrupt the delicate balance of the human microbiome and interfere with hormonal functions, potentially igniting inflammatory responses. The choice between organic and nonorganic foods, then, becomes not just a matter of nutritional content but also of weighing the invisible costs of chemical exposure against the benefits of reduced pesticide intake. In foods known to have high pesticide residues—such as strawberries, spinach, and apples—the shift towards organic is a strategic move to minimize inflammatory triggers.

Empowerment for food choices begins with education, transforming you from a passive participant to an informed advocate for your health. This empowerment is rooted in an understanding of ingredient lists and nutrition facts, alongside recognizing the inflammatory catalysts hidden within. It involves not just scanning for familiar culprits but also developing an awareness of serving sizes, sugar content, and the types of fats present.

Trans fats, for instance, are notorious for their inflammatory properties and may still be found in trace amounts under the guise of "partially hydrogenated oils" despite widespread bans. Similarly, the sugars that fuel inflammation may proliferate under various names: fructose, sucrose, corn syrup—each a different mask for the same inflammatory potential.

Our choice of foods involves an act of discernment—a balance between the pleasures of taste and the pursuit of health. It calls for a shift from passive consumption to active engagement—from accepting labels at face value to questioning and uncovering the truths they may conceal. This shift does not demand perfection but rather an orientation towards mindfulness and a willingness to look beyond the surface and make choices that align with your deeper goals of health and well-being.

Ultimately, decoding food labels embodies a broader commitment to self-care, nurturing the body with foods that heal rather than harm. It reflects a conscious decision to engage with your food not as a bystander but as an informed participant armed with knowledge and driven by the conviction that the foods you choose have the power to shape your health and your response to inflammation.

In this endeavor, every label decoded, additive identified, and mindful choice made contributes to a larger tapestry of health woven one food choice at a time.

Inflammation and Chronic Diseases:

Understanding the Link

Chronic inflammation is often subtle yet pervasive, weaving a way to numerous diseases that often go unnoticed until a pattern of illness becomes unmistakable. This insidious process has a hand in the genesis and progression of conditions as varied as arthritis, heart disease, and diabetes—diseases that, at first glance, seem to share little beyond their chronic nature; yet, at their core, they reveal a common antagonist: an immune system stuck in relentless, misguided action against the body it was designed to protect.

The link between chronic inflammation and such diseases is not merely one of correlation but causation. In arthritis, the visuals are stark: joints swollen, mobility compromised—the result of an immune system attacking the very tissues it should safeguard. This condition serves as a vivid illustration of inflammation's potential to become harmful when its regulatory mechanisms falter, consequently turning self-defense into self-destruction.

With heart disease, the connection unfolds more subtly. Here, inflammation acts not with the overt aggression seen in arthritis but as a silent accomplice to atherosclerosis—where arterial walls thicken not from injury but from the accumulation of fatty deposits ensnared in a web of inflammatory cells. The gradual, cumulative damage leads to heart attacks and strokes that seemingly strike without warning.

Diabetes, particularly type-2, further exemplifies the intricate dance between inflammation and chronic disease. The condition begins not with a sudden failure of the pancreas but with insulin resistance—a state wherein cells besieged by inflammatory signals no longer respond to insulin's attempts to regulate blood sugar levels. The pancreas attempts, in vain, to compensate by producing more insulin. Blood sugar rises, and diabetes ensues—a testament to inflammation's role in disrupting the body's metabolic harmony.

Against this backdrop of disease, diet emerges as a powerful mediator—a means of influencing the inflammatory process for better or worse. The foods we consume can either fuel or quell inflammation, depending on whether they're high in refined sugars and unhealthy fats or rich in omega-3 fatty acids, antioxidants, and phytonutrients, respectively. An anti-inflammatory diet—rich in fruits, vegetables, whole grains, and lean proteins—does more than nourish; it's also an immune system modulator, as it dampens the flames of inflammation and thus reduces the risk of the diseases it engenders.

Yet, diet is only one piece of the puzzle. Other lifestyle factors play critical roles in either exacerbating or alleviating inflammation. For instance, stress acts as a trigger for the release of cortisol—a hormone that, in excess, promotes inflammation. The modern world, with its relentless pace and pressures, is a veritable breeding ground for stress, therefore making stress management not just beneficial but also necessary for quelling chronic inflammation. Techniques such as mindfulness meditation, deep breathing exercises, and yoga offer refuge and tools to calm the mind and, by extension, the body.

Sleep, too, holds sway over inflammation. The restorative power of sleep is well-documented, as it's a time when the body repairs and regenerates—processes that chronic inflammation can largely disrupt, creating a negative feedback loop of unrestful sleep and increased inflammation. In the absence of adequate sleep, the body is deprived of its full complement of restorative cycles and enters a state of low-grade inflammation, setting the stage for the development and progression of chronic diseases. Thus, prioritizing sleep—ensuring both quantity and quality—is a vital strategy in managing inflammation.

Exercise completes this triad of lifestyle factors influencing inflammation. Its benefits extend beyond cardiovascular health and weight management and reach into the realm of inflammatory responses. Regular, moderate exercise has been shown to reduce inflammatory markers and thus enhance immune function and metabolic health. The key lies in consistency and moderation. You can engage in walking, cycling, swimming, or any activity that elevates your heart rate and invigorates your body; just make sure that it's both enjoyable and sustainable.

The actionable steps to mitigate the risk of chronic inflammatory diseases through diet and lifestyle changes are clear. They begin with dietary adjustments to incorporate anti-inflammatory foods and reduce or eliminate those that promote inflammation. They also extend into the realms of stress management, sleep optimization, and regular physical activity—each a pillar supporting your long-term health.

Together, these strategies form a comprehensive approach to reducing inflammation that acknowledges the complexity of our bodies' systems and the myriad ways in which we can influence our health outcomes. Through informed choices and deliberate actions, we can modulate inflammation, steering our health trajectories away from chronic disease and toward vitality and longevity.

Chapter 2:

Quenching Flames—Foods That Cool Down Inflammation

Chronic inflammation is often a persistent antagonist in the narrative of well-being that doesn't discriminate, silently and inadvertently impacting our entire lives. Our diet's role in preventing and mitigating these impacts cannot be overstated; what we choose to eat can either fan the flames of inflammation or help extinguish them. This chapter turns the spotlight on the dietary heroes of the fight against inflammation. First, we'll take a look at the potent anti-inflammatory effects of omega-3 fatty acids.

Omega-3 Rich Foods: Your Best Allies

Health Benefits of Omega-3s

Omega-3 fatty acids are a type of unsaturated fat, and they have garnered acclaim for their anti-inflammatory prowess. These essential fats—so named because the body cannot produce them independently—play a critical role in cellular function and our overall health. They're known to mitigate inflammation by interfering with the production of inflammatory compounds such as eicosanoids and cytokines. The benefits of omega-3s extend beyond inflammation, however; research suggests a link between omega-3 consumption and a reduced risk of heart disease, support for mental health, and alleviation of autoimmune conditions (NIH, 2023).

Sources of Omega-3s

Omega-3 fatty acids are found in both animal and plant sources, each offering a different form of this essential nutrient. Oily fish such as salmon, mackerel, and sardines are rich in eicosapentaenoic acid (EPA) and docosahexaenoic acid (DHA)—omega-3s that the body can readily use. For those who prefer plant-based sources, flaxseeds, chia seeds, and walnuts provide alpha-linoleic acid (ALA), which the body can partially convert to EPA and DHA. Including a variety of these sources in your diet ensures a broad spectrum of omega-3 benefits.

Incorporating Omega-3s Into Meals

Integrating omega-3-rich foods into your daily meals requires a blend of creativity and intention. You could start the day with a chia seed pudding or add ground flaxseeds to your morning oatmeal for a plant-based omega-3 boost. For lunch or dinner, grilled salmon or mackerel can serve as the centerpiece of a meal rich in both flavor and nutrients. You can also choose to snack on a handful of walnuts or enrich your salads with a flaxseed oil dressing to effortlessly increase your omega-3 intake. The goal is to make omega-3s a consistent part of your diet.

Supplementation

While food sources are the preferred method for obtaining omega-3s, supplements can play a role in bridging nutritional gaps, especially for individuals with specific health concerns or dietary restrictions. When considering supplementation, look for high-quality fish, krill, or algal oil (a plant-based option) that provides both EPA and DHA in concentrations sufficient to impact health. Consult with a healthcare provider to determine the appropriate dosage for your body and ensure that supplements complement rather than conflict with your health regimen.

Visual Element: Omega-3 Rich Foods Infographic

To make it as easy as possible for you to incorporate omega-3 fatty acids into your diet, try putting together "Your Omega-3 Toolkit," visually presenting a selection of both animal-based and plant-based omega-3 sources, their serving sizes, and the approximate omega-3 content in each. This visual guide will ensure that you can easily take a well-rounded approach to fighting inflammation by serving as a quick reference for a diverse range of sources of omega-3s to choose from.

In the ongoing battle against chronic inflammation, the dietary choices we make can significantly sway the tide in our favor. With their robust anti-inflammatory properties, omega-3 fatty acids are powerful allies in this fight. By prioritizing these essential fats in our diet, we harness a natural strategy to quell inflammation, protect our health, and enhance our quality of life. Navigating the complexities of nutritional health toward choices that foster well-being involves letting our knowledge of omega-3s guide us, one meal at a time.

Colorful Vegetables: The More, the Merrier

Vegetables offer not only a wealth of vibrant hues that can help make our plates more visually appealing, but they also contain a plethora of nutrients beneath their skins. Their kaleidoscope of colors does more than please the eye; it serves as a code, with each shade indicating an array of phytonutrients and antioxidants that arm the body against the insidious creep of inflammation.

The significance of plant compounds in combating inflammation cannot be overstated. They operate on a cellular level, neutralizing free radicals and thus thwarting the oxidative stress that often precedes inflammation. Moreover, the diversity of phytonutrients found across the spectrum of vegetables ensures a comprehensive approach to inflammation by addressing different pathways through which inflammation can manifest.

Ensuring variety in your vegetable consumption allows these compounds to work in synergy. No single vegetable can claim to hold a cure for inflammation; rather, it's in the collective, broad palette of vegetables consumed that their true strength lies. This diversity ensures a broad coverage of nutrients, effectively creating interlocking shields of protection against inflammation. From the deep purples of eggplants that are rich in nasunin to the bright oranges of carrots, laden with beta-carotene, each vegetable contributes a unique set of phytochemicals that can collectively fortify your body's defenses.

Just as with the varying sources of omega-3s, expanding the repertoire of vegetables in your daily meals requires both creativity and intention. It starts with breakfast, where spinach or kale can transform your ordinary omelet into a nutrient-dense start to the day. Lunch and dinner present further opportunities, with salads offering flexible opportunities for a medley of vegetables, grains, and proteins dressed with olive oil-based vinaigrettes that complement the anti-inflammatory theme. Snacks need not be left out of this colorful revolution either; crudité platters turn raw vegetables into convenient "munchables" that can be paired with hummus or guacamole for added flavor and nutrients. Even desserts can partake, with zucchini bread or beet-based chocolate cake offering you a sweet yet healthful indulgence.

Embracing seasonal eating further amplifies the benefits of a vegetable-rich diet, subsequently aligning the body's needs with the rhythms of nature. This practice not only maximizes the nutrient intake you can get from vegetables—harvested at their peak of ripeness—but also contributes to environmental sustainability by reducing the demand for out-of-season produce that often has a heavier carbon footprint due to transportation from distant locales.

Additionally, following the seasonal cycle offers natural diversity by encouraging a rotation of vegetables in your diet and thus preventing nutritional monotony. Spring brings leafy greens such as arugula and Swiss chard; summer offers a bounty of tomatoes and bell peppers; fall introduces the richness of squashes and pumpkins; and winter provides hearty root vegetables like turnips and parsnips. This cyclical dietary pattern not only nurtures the body with seasonal nutrients but also fosters a connection with the local environment and its agricultural rhythms.

Vegetables play a pivotal role in any anti-inflammatory diet, and their colors are a guide to the nutrients within. By adopting a diverse, vegetable-rich diet—anchored in the principles of phytonutrient variety and seasonal eating—you can take a strategic approach to mitigating inflammation. This approach calls for a shift in perception: View every meal as an opportunity to nourish and protect your body with the vibrant bounty of the earth. This subtle yet profound shift holds the promise of transforming your health—one colorful vegetable at a time.

Spices and Herbs: Nature's Anti-Inflammatory Agents

When culinary mastery meets health science, the power of spices and herbs extends far beyond their modest quantities. These botanical treasures not only add flavor but also significantly dampen the fires of inflammation. Among the plethora of options, turmeric and ginger are exemplars of nature's capacity to provide relief and promote healing through dietary means. With its vibrant golden hue, turmeric owes its anti-inflammatory prowess to curcumin—a compound that research has shown to rival over-the-counter remedies in its ability to provide anti-inflammatory respite without adverse effects. Ginger operates similarly with the compound gingerol acting as the main bioactive component responsible for its powerful anti-inflammatory and antioxidant effects.

The list of herbs that can contribute to your anti-inflammatory arsenal is extensive: Basil's aromatic leaves contain eugenol, which mirrors the anti-inflammatory properties of over-the-counter pain medication. Oregano and thyme are rich in carvacrol and thymol, respectively, and they share a capacity to interrupt the synthesis of inflammation-promoting enzymes, hence offering a culinary strategy for mitigating discomfort. When integrated into daily meals, these herbs work synergistically with the body's natural processes to reduce inflammation and promote well-being.

Incorporating these potent ingredients into everyday cooking begins with the recognition of the power held in each pinch and dash. The incorporation of turmeric into morning smoothies or the inclusion of a ginger infusion in your evening teas are simple yet profound acts of self-care. Herbs like basil and oregano find their place in sauces and dressings, thus transforming mundane dishes into experiences that are not only rich and flavorful but also soothing and healing. The approach here is not about overhauling your diet but, rather, gradually integrating the spices and herbs that offer the most potent anti-inflammatory benefits in a way that you can enjoy.

The creation of DIY seasoning blends can empower you to harness the full spectrum of flavors and health benefits these ingredients offer. A simple blend might combine turmeric, black pepper (which enhances curcumin absorption), ginger, and garlic powder to create a versatile seasoning that can be applied to proteins, vegetables, or grains. A Mediterranean-style anti-inflammatory blend might feature basil, oregano, thyme, and rosemary. These homemade concoctions not only elevate the culinary experience but also imbue everyday meals with their healing and protecting capacity.

The interplay between our diet and our health is complex and nuanced, varying according to each of our individual needs and responses. Yet, spices and herbs stand out for their universal applicability and profound impact. Their incorporation into your diet combines pleasure and health in a marriage of the sensory and the medicinal. In this light, the kitchen transforms from a place of mere sustenance to a sanctuary of healing, where each ingredient chosen and each meal prepared is imbued with your intention to improve your overall health.

This approach to cooking and eating is not merely about adding flavor or following recipes; it's an acknowledgment of the power that food has to influence your health—one that can be magnified by selecting ingredients with therapeutic properties. With their concentrated compounds, herbs and spices offer a direct line to leveraging this power. They remind us that healing is not always a matter of pharmaceuticals or interventions; it can begin on our plates with the choices we make at each meal.

In this way, the act of cooking becomes an act of care—a daily opportunity to nourish your body as a whole, starting from the very cells and physiological mechanisms that sustain it. Over time, this practice can shift the balance of your health toward vitality by reducing inflammation. Through this lens, the inclusion of anti-inflammatory spices and herbs in our diet can be seen as not just a culinary choice but also a holistic strategy for living well.

The Power of Berries: Small but Mighty

The diminutive size of berries belies their dense concentration of antioxidants—vigilant protectors that patrol the body's cellular pathways seeking out and neutralizing the free radicals that, if left unchecked, contribute to the cascade of inflammation. This section takes a closer look at these potent botanicals by exploring the diversity of berries available, elucidating simple yet effective methods for their incorporation into your daily eating patterns, and navigating the debate between the virtues of fresh versus frozen varieties.

The antioxidant capacity of berries is a key feature that positions these fruits as essential players in an anti-inflammatory diet. Antioxidants such as vitamin C, flavonoids, and anthocyanins are abundant in berries, each contributing to the mitigation of oxidative stress and, consequently, the reduction of inflammation. Scientific investigations into the effects of these compounds reveal a consistent pattern: Regular consumption of berries is linked with a decrease in markers of inflammation, therefore suggesting a protective effect that extends beyond the gut, influences systemic health, and potentially lowers the risk of various chronic diseases.

The assortment of available berries is vast, encompassing both the familiar and the exotic. Strawberries and blueberries are staples in many diets and are renowned not only for their versatility and palatability but also for their rich anthocyanin content, which imparts both vivid coloration and robust antioxidant properties. With a delicate structure and tangy flavor, raspberries offer a bounty of fiber and vitamin C, while dense and dark blackberries are laden with vitamins, minerals, and antioxidants. On the more exotic end of the spectrum, goji and acai berries offer unique nutritional profiles; the former is prized for its high vitamin C and zeaxanthin content, the latter for its heart-healthy fats and anthocyanins. Each variety of berry brings its own set of benefits, suggesting that diversity in berry consumption can maximize the anti-inflammatory potential of one's diet.

Incorporating berries into your meals and snacks doesn't demand any culinary expertise but rather a willingness to experiment and explore. Starting the day with a smoothie enriched with a mix of berries could provide you with an early morning antioxidant boost. For snacks, you may want to try a handful of mixed berries, offering a refreshing, nutrient-dense alternative to processed options. Berries can also transform salads from mundane to extraordinary by adding a burst of flavor and color that enhances both the aesthetic and nutritional value of the dish. Your desserts, too, can hugely benefit from the inclusion of berries; a simple berry compote over yogurt or spread on whole-grain pancakes can satisfy sweet cravings while contributing to the body's anti-inflammatory arsenal.

The choice between fresh and frozen berries is more than a matter of convenience; it touches upon considerations of nutritional integrity and availability. The prevailing assumption that fresh is always better doesn't hold firm under scrutiny, however. Studies indicate that frozen berries—picked at their peak ripeness and immediately frozen—can not only preserve but also surpass the antioxidant capacity of their fresh counterparts, which may lose nutritional value during transport and storage (Brown, 2017). The key to enjoying a potentially superior year-round source of antioxidants lies in selecting frozen berries that are free from added sugars or preservatives, hence ensuring that the nutritional benefits aren't undermined by unnecessary additives.

In combating inflammation, berries emerge as champion fruits for their dense nutritional content, diverse variety, and versatile use in culinary creations. The evidence in favor of regular berry consumption is compelling, thereby positioning these small but mighty fruits as valuable allies in the quest for optimal health. Through strategic incorporation into your diet, berries, whether fresh or frozen, can contribute significantly to your body's defense against inflammation, offering a delicious and accessible means to support your well-being.

Nuts and Seeds: Snacks That Fight Inflammation

Nuts and seeds are diminutive powerhouses that are often overlooked in their contribution to health. They pack a dense nutritional punch by offering a powerful combination of fats, proteins, vitamins, and minerals that collectively fortify the body's defenses against the insidious creep of inflammation. In the modern dietary landscape, the prevalence of processed foods has largely led to an imbalance in the types of fats consumed, pushing many of us toward an inflammatory state. In this context, nuts and seeds offer a path to return to equilibrium—a means to rebalance your diet in favor of wellness.

The way we think of dietary fats has long been dominated by a dichotomy between the virtues of their nutrients and the vilification of their caloric content. Yet, this binary fails to capture the nuance of the role these fats play in health and inflammation. While it's true that an excessive intake of saturated fats—particularly from processed sources—can promote inflammation, these fats are not inherently detrimental when eaten in moderation. In fact, fats, as a whole, are essential and play distinct roles in bodily functions; the solution lies in the ratio of various fatty acids within our diets. Modern eating habits have skewed this ratio heavily in favor of omega-6 fats, thus, disrupting the delicate balance required for optimal health. This is where nuts and seeds come in: For instance, the omega-3 content of walnuts offers a counterpoint to the omega-6 dominance in typical diets. Similarly, flaxseeds and chia seeds provide ALA—a plant-based omega-3 fat— further contributing to the dietary equilibrium between these essential fats.

Besides their omega-3 content, the vitamin E and selenium found in almonds and Brazil nuts, respectively, reduce oxidative stress and inflammation by neutralizing free radicals The collective intake of a variety of nuts and seeds ensures a comprehensive approach to inflammation, thereby leveraging the full spectrum of their health benefits.

Integrating nuts and seeds into your diet transcends the simplicity of snacking on a handful of these morsels; it invites you to reimagine their role in your daily eating patterns by encouraging innovative uses that enhance both flavor and nutritional value. You can choose to enrich your smoothie with a spoonful of ground flaxseed, or sprinkle sunflower seeds onto your midday salad to add crunch and substance. The versatility of nuts and seeds extends into baking, where almond flour offers a nutrient-dense gluten-free alternative to traditional wheat flour, and pumpkin seeds can add texture and nutrients to breads and muffins. Even in the realm of desserts, you can find varied uses for these nutrition boosters: A crust of mixed nuts for a pie or a garnish of toasted sesame seeds on a batch of homemade granola bars demonstrates the creative potential of these ingredients.

Nuts and seeds can work to not only satisfy hunger but also contribute to your body's overall well-being. Every food choice you make offers an opportunity to support healing and wellness, and with this in mind, you can see that nuts and seeds are not merely snacks but integral components of a dietary strategy aimed at reducing inflammation and enhancing your quality of life. Through conscious choices and creative culinary applications, these natural treasures can play a pivotal role in a holistic approach to health—one that embraces the complexity of nutrition and its impact on your body's intricate systems.

Legumes and Whole Grains: Fiber-Rich Foods for Gut Health

The fiber found in legumes and whole grains acts not merely as a digestive aid but also as a prebiotic nourishing the beneficial bacteria that colonize the gut and form the first line of defense against inflammatory processes. This relationship between a well-nourished microbiome and reduced inflammation underscores the critical role that legumes and whole grains occupy as bastions of gut health, protecting against incursions of inflammation.

Selecting the most effective types of legumes and whole grains for an anti-inflammatory diet requires a discerning eye: For legumes, this means gravitating towards varieties such as lentils, garbanzo beans, and black beans, which are not only versatile in their culinary uses but also particularly rich in soluble fiber and resistant starches. Their fermentation in the colon produces short-chain fatty acids that can strengthen your gut barrier and reduce inflammation. It is also important to carefully examine which "whole" grains are, indeed, *whole*. True whole grains—including quinoa, barley, and brown rice—retain all parts of the grain kernel, therefore providing a full spectrum of anti-inflammatory nutrients including B vitamins and minerals.

The seemingly mundane culinary preparation of legumes and whole grains is actually crucial when it comes to maximizing their nutritional profile and digestibility. Soaking your legumes in water, for instance, reduces their phytic acid levels and makes their minerals more bioavailable, consequently enhancing their anti-inflammatory potential. Cooking methods also matter: Simmering legumes at a gentle boil can preserve the integrity of their nutrients; steaming or boiling whole grains can retain their nutritional content without introducing unhealthy additives. The ancient technique of sprouting can further increase legumes' antioxidant levels, thus amplifying their roles as anti-inflammatory agents.

Transforming these humble ingredients into dishes that delight your palate while nourishing your body offers a canvas for culinary creativity. Their hearty textures can anchor a meal by serving as the foundation for soups, stews, or salads or being transformed into nutritious yet savory spreads and dips. When the nutty flavors and satisfying chew of whole grains are paired with a wide array of vegetables, proteins, and healthy fats, they create a versatile base for bowls, pilafs, and even breakfast porridges. Think of the integration of these foods as an opportunity to support your gut health and, by extension, combat inflammation.

Including legumes and whole grains is a dietary strategy that leans on the foundational elements of fiber and nutrients to build a defense against the pervasive threat of inflammation. Every choice matters— from the selection of the most nutrient-dense options to the methods of preparation and integration into daily meals. This is a strategy that doesn't seek to overhaul your dietary habits with drastic changes but instead weave the threads of gut-friendly anti-inflammatory foods into the fabric of your everyday eating practices.

In this chapter, we've traced the paths by which these fiber- and nutrient-rich foods can nourish your gut microbiome, strengthen your gut barrier, and reduce your body's inflammatory processes. In doing so, we've illuminated the broader principle that underpins an anti-inflammatory diet: Food, in its most natural and least processed form, harbors the potential to not only nourish but also heal. Though this is simple in its essence, it offers an invitation to reconsider your dietary choices and make a shift towards foods that support your body's natural defenses against inflammation. As we turn the page, this principle guides us forward, leading us deeper into the exploration of dietary strategies that harness the power of food to enhance health and well-being.

Chapter 3:

Crafting an Anti-Inflammatory

Blueprint

The art of meal planning requires both foresight and creativity. It's not simply about filling a plate; it's about curating a selection of foods that work in harmony to nourish and protect the body. This chapter delves into the practical aspects of constructing a meal plan that aligns with anti-inflammatory principles and guides readers through setting personal health goals, balancing meal components, and strategizing weekly meal preparation.

Crafting Your Anti-Inflammatory Meal Plan

Setting Goals and Preferences

Before a painter touches their brush to any canvas, they must first envision what they seek to create. Similarly, defining health goals and dietary preferences forms the initial step in meal planning. This process involves a clear assessment of current health conditions, dietary restrictions, and personal taste preferences. For someone with arthritis, the goal might focus on reducing joint inflammation and pain, consequently necessitating a diet low in sugar and saturated fats but rich in omega-3 fatty acids. Likewise, someone looking to improve gut health might prioritize fiber-rich foods that support a healthy microbiome. This phase of planning is deeply personal and sets the foundation for a meal plan that not only addresses your specific health objectives but also aligns with your individual tastes, ensuring both sustainability and enjoyment. For instance, one of my favorite meals is a three-bean chili that is not only delicious but also packed with protein, fiber, and essential vitamins and minerals. It can also be served over brown rice, in a whole-grain tortilla, or with corn chips, allowing for lots of variety with little extra effort.

Balanced Meal Components

In a well-constructed meal, each component plays a critical role in achieving dietary harmony. This balance involves a careful selection of macronutrients—carbohydrates, proteins, and fats—combined with a rich array of vitamins and minerals derived from fruits, vegetables, nuts, seeds, and spices. Each meal should aim to include a source of lean protein to support tissue repair and growth, whether from an animal source like salmon or plant-based like lentils. You can choose carbohydrates from whole grains and vegetables for fiber and essential nutrients. Omega-3s from, for instance, flaxseeds or walnuts can round out your meal, improve cellular health, and reduce inflammation. By considering the inflammatory or anti-inflammatory properties of your foods, you can construct meals that not only satisfy your hunger but also actively contribute to your health goals.

Weekly Planning Strategies

A quote that is often attributed to Benjamin Franklin states, "By failing to prepare, you are preparing to fail," and that aptly applies to meal planning. Effectively strategizing for a week of anti-inflammatory eating involves drafting a meal plan, creating a detailed shopping list, and setting aside time for meal prep. This process begins with selecting recipes that fit the week's objectives taking into account your financial and time constraints, the seasonal availability of ingredients, and variety to prevent boredom. Next, compiling a shopping list organized by department or aisle—by categorizing items as produce, dairy, meats, or dry goods—can streamline the shopping experience, consequently making you more efficient and less prone to impulse purchases that deviate from the plan. Finally, designating a meal prep day—often a weekend afternoon—allows for the bulk preparation of ingredients ranging from chopping vegetables to cooking grains and even assembling full meals that require only reheating. This approach not only saves time during the busy workweek but also ensures that healthy, anti-inflammatory meals are always within reach.

Sample Meal Plans

To bridge the gap between theory and practice, you can create a series of sample meal plans, each designed to cater to your dietary preferences and health goals. By preparing these in advance, you provide yourself with an easy path to making effective choices in the future by streamlining the decision-making process. This allows you to truly focus on meal preparation, rather than planning, in the first few weeks of implementing the change to an anti-inflammatory diet.

One such plan might feature oatmeal topped with berries and chia seeds for breakfast; a quinoa salad with roasted vegetables and garbanzo beans for lunch; and baked salmon with steamed broccoli and sweet potato for dinner. Snacks could include sliced apples with almond butter or a handful of mixed nuts. Each meal and snack should be selected for its nutrient profile while focusing on anti-inflammatory benefits. Once you have prepared these templates based on your needs and preferences, they will serve as a starting point encouraging you to adopt an anti-inflammatory diet.

Visual Element: Weekly Meal Plan Template

It can be hugely helpful to seek out a downloadable template for a weekly meal plan that features sections for breakfast, lunch, dinner, and snacks for each day of the week. These tools are designed to help you organize your meal-planning process by allowing for easy customization and adjustments based on your specific goals and preferences. They also tend to include a shopping list section organized by food categories to assist in efficient grocery shopping. If you are digitally savvy and like to rely on online recipes, many meal plan templates can even auto-compile your shopping list when you insert the URLs of the recipes you'll be using.

I found this incredibly beneficial when initially making changes to my diet, as it meant that I could devote less of my mental energy to the planning stage and therefore have more to devote to experimenting with new foods and cooking methods.

Shopping List Essentials: Building an Anti-Inflammatory Pantry

As we aim to not just manage but actively discourage inflammation, our pantries become a crucial battlefield. On your shelves and within your drawers lies the potential for both harm and healing depending on the arsenal of ingredients at your disposal.

The construction of an anti-inflammatory pantry is not merely about stocking up on beneficial foods but about creating a repository of nutritional tools that can be wielded with precision to combat inflammation at its roots. This meticulous assembly of pantry staples is the first step in transforming your kitchen from a place of sustenance to a sanctuary of health.

Pantry Staples

The cornerstone of an anti-inflammatory pantry are items that warrant a permanent space on your shelves due to their versatility and health benefits:

- With its heart-healthy monounsaturated fats and polyphenols, extra-virgin olive oil can serve as your primary cooking fat replacing more inflammatory options like vegetable oils.

- Whole grains like quinoa, farro, and brown rice offer fiber and essential nutrients while serving as foundational elements for a multitude of dishes.

- Seeds and nuts—including flaxseeds, chia seeds, almonds, and walnuts—are not just snacks but also sources of omega-3s and antioxidants.

- From lentils to garbanzo beans, legumes provide plant-based protein and fiber essential for gut health and inflammation control.

- Spices and herbs—particularly turmeric, ginger, basil, and oregano—can also be kept on hand to transform your meals into anti-inflammatory feasts with their potent phytochemicals.

This curated selection ensures that the building blocks for healthful meals are always within reach, ready to be transformed into dishes that nourish both your body and soul.

Smart Shopping Tips

Navigating the aisles of grocery stores and markets requires not just a list but a strategy—an approach that prioritizes quality and nutritional value while avoiding the pitfalls of marketing and convenience:

- Focus on fresh produce, meats, dairy, and whenever possible, choose organic options to reduce exposure to inflammatory pesticides and antibiotics.

- Bypass processed foods in favor of whole, minimally processed alternatives.

- Bulk buying sections offer an opportunity to purchase staples like grains, nuts, and seeds at a lower cost.

- Familiarity with seasonal produce can also guide shopping choices and synchronize purchases with the rhythms of nature for maximum nutritional benefit.

This mindful approach to shopping reinforces your commitment to an anti-inflammatory lifestyle.

Budget-Friendly Choices

Adhering to an anti-inflammatory diet need not strain your finances; it only necessitates a thoughtful allocation of resources. Prioritizing your expenditure begins with seeking out sales and discounts on the essential items that form the backbone of an anti-inflammatory diet. Investing in quality pivotal items—such as olive oil and organic produce—will save you from compromising on nutrients critical for inflammation control. For items with a longer shelf life, such as grains and legumes, bulk purchases can offer significant savings. You can also alleviate budgetary pressures by incorporating more plant-based proteins in your diet, as they are generally less expensive than their animal-based counterparts. This judicious approach to spending ensures that your pursuit of health is sustainable, both nutritionally and financially.

Storing Essentials

Proper storage preserves both nutritional value and flavor. Whole grains and legumes are susceptible to spoilage when exposed to moisture and air, so they benefit from airtight containers and a cool, dark environment. The high oil content in nuts and seeds can sometimes entail refrigerator or freezer storage to prevent rancidity, extend their shelf life, and preserve their health benefits. Spices and herbs, though more durable, also require protection from light and heat to maintain their potency. Likewise, olive oil thrives in a dark, cool space; its container should be well-sealed to guard against oxidation.

This careful protection of your ingredients not only extends their usability but also ensures that their anti-inflammatory properties are preserved, ready to be unleashed in the service of your health. The battle against inflammation is fought and won in the kitchen—one ingredient, one dish, and one day at a time.

Meal Prep 101: Tips for Busy Individuals

In contemporary life, each day unfurls with its own set of demands, and hours seem to slip through our fingers like grains of sand. As a result, the act of meal preparation is not a mere culinary endeavor but rather a strategic exercise in time management and stress reduction. The art of meal prepping, therefore, is not just about assembling ingredients but about implementing efficiency that aligns with the demands of your daily commitments. This section offers insights into methods that streamline the cooking process and ensure that nourishment and convenience coalesce in every dish.

Efficient Meal Prep Techniques

Aiming for efficiency in meal preparation guides the way toward techniques that condense hours of cooking into manageable intervals of focused activity. This process begins with the segregation of tasks according to their nature and complexity.

For instance, with their varied forms and textures, vegetables demand an approach that respects their individual requirements. Washing, drying, chopping, and storing them in clear, labeled containers sets the stage for their seamless integration into meals; but some veggies, like peppers, lose a lot of their vitamin C content once cut and exposed to oxygen, so these may need to be frozen or cooked and integrated into dishes during meal prep to maintain their nutritional benefits. Proteins, whether plant-based or animal-derived, benefit from marinating in advance—a step that imbues them with flavor while tenderizing their structures.

Grains and legumes can be cooked in large quantities and portioned for subsequent meals, ready to be imbued with the colors and tastes of accompanying ingredients. Through these methods, the foundation for a week of nutritious eating is laid, with each step designed to make the most of your time and create pockets of opportunity for healthful eating.

Batch Cooking

Batch cooking recognizes that today's efforts can bear fruit in the days to follow. This approach hinges on the principle of scalability— i.e., leveraging the same amount of kitchen time to produce multiple servings of a dish that can be enjoyed throughout the week. Soups, stews, casseroles, and curries lend themselves admirably to this technique as their flavors deepen with time, transforming leftovers into sought-after treasures. The strategic selection of dishes that freeze well expands this horizon further, thus ensuring that a reservoir of healthy meals stands ready to meet your future dietary needs without sacrificing quality or taste. This helps you resist the temptation to resort to less healthful, convenient options.

Prep and Store

The transition from preparation to consumption is bridged by the critical phase of storage—a step that safeguards the freshness and nutritional integrity of prepped ingredients and meals. The inert nature and transparency of glass containers allow for easy identification of contents, and their airtight seals preserve the flavors and textures within. The allocation of your refrigerator and freezer space should follow a system that prioritizes accessibility and rotation, thus ensuring that the most perishable items are used first and that each meal is as vibrant and nourishing as intended. This meticulous organization extends the lifespan of ingredients, reduces waste, and maintains a steady supply of anti-inflammatory foods.

Quick and Healthy Meal Ideas

Quick and healthy recipes transform prepped ingredients into culinary delights with minimal additional effort. A base of mixed greens can be topped with pre-roasted vegetables, a sprinkle of seeds or nuts, and slices of grilled chicken or marinated tofu, all dressed in a homemade vinaigrette that was whisked together during meal prep. You can reclaim your right to an unhurried breakfast with overnight oats in pre-assembled jars. Even snacks can be elevated from mere afterthoughts to deliberate choices that sustain energy and curb inflammation; hummus with sliced vegetables or apple rounds with almond butter provide quick, satisfying options that align with the broader objectives of health and well-being. Indeed, meal prepping offers a mosaic of flavors and nutrients that can support your body's fight against inflammation while respecting the constraints of time.

The strategic embrace of meal prep offers hope and a path to success when the demands of work, family, and personal pursuits collide. This preparation becomes a ritual of empowerment and a daily reaffirmation of your commitment to a lifestyle that values nourishment, mindfulness, and the profound impact of diet on well-being.

Reading and Understanding Nutritional Information

The ability to decode nutrition labels is a pivotal skill that equips you with the discernment to distinguish between foods that heal and those that harm. Packaged foods, in particular, are often a minefield of hidden inflammatory agents masquerading under the guise of health, so they demand a keen eye and an informed mind. This section will arm you with the tools necessary to peel back the layers of marketing and reveal the core nutritional truths of the foods you consume, thereby ensuring every choice you make can contribute to your overarching health goals.

Understanding the Challenges of Nutrition Labels

Although the nutritional lexicon is standardized, it often confounds with its density of information. At its heart, a nutrition label provides a snapshot of a food's nutritional value, detailing macronutrients—fats, proteins, and carbohydrates—and micronutrients—vitamins and minerals. Yet, beyond these basics lies a deeper narrative of serving sizes and percentages of daily values—metrics that offer context but can mislead without proper understanding. For instance, a serving size determined by the manufacturer of a food may be chosen to downplay its caloric content and not align with realistic consumption patterns, consequently skewing your perception of the nutrients ingested. Similarly, the daily value percentages provided on labels are based on a generalized 2,000-calorie diet, and they may not reflect your individual nutritional needs, thus necessitating adjustments based on your specific health goals and dietary requirements.

Identifying Key Nutrients

Certain nutrients have anti-inflammatory potential that can guide your choices toward foods that dampen inflammation's flames. As we discussed in Chapter 2, for example, omega-3 fatty acids are heralded for their capacity to reduce inflammatory markers—a trait not often explicitly listed but inferred from the presence of fish oils or flaxseeds in the ingredient list. Fiber is another ally that exerts its effects indirectly by fostering a gut environment conducive to anti-inflammatory microbial communities; its presence is often explicitly listed on nutritional labels. Antioxidants, though a diverse group, share the common trait of combating oxidative stress—a precursor to inflammation. The inclusion of vitamins C and E, along with selenium and zinc, serve as indicators of antioxidant-rich foods. Understanding these key nutrients and their roles in the anti-inflammatory process transforms the act of reading a nutrition label from a routine task into a strategic, proactive decision-making process supportive of your health.

Portion Sizes and Servings

Balancing portion sizes and servings is a critical aspect of managing an anti-inflammatory diet that ensures the body receives what it needs without tipping the scales toward inflammation. Your body's needs aren't static; they fluctuate based on your activity levels, metabolic health, and even circadian rhythm. Thus, portion control—informed by an understanding of the nutritional content of your foods and your current needs—is an effective tool in modulating inflammation.

Avoiding Marketing Traps

The ability to distinguish genuine nutritional merit from the allure of marketing claims is what sets those who navigate their food choices with confidence apart from those ensnared by dietary illusions. Health claims, though regulated and technically accurate, often skirt the boundaries of truth offering promises that may not hold significance in the context of an anti-inflammatory diet. Terms like "low-fat" or "high in fiber" may conceal the presence of sugars, sodium, or artificial additives that negate any potential benefits.

Thankfully, you can learn to look beyond these claims; assess foods based on their comprehensive nutritional profile and ingredient composition; and favor whole, minimally processed, anti-inflammatory options. This discernment is grounded in knowledge and honed through practice and it can empower you to make choices that truly serve your health—selections that support your journey to well-being with every bite taken.

The mastery of nutritional information demands diligence, patience, and a commitment to learning—traits that, once cultivated, become second nature and guide dietary choices with an informed grace that ensures every decision is made in the service of health.

Substitutions for Common Inflammatory Ingredients

The act of substitution involves precision and innovation that is tuned in to the symphony of flavors that define a dish. To navigate an anti-inflammatory diet requires a deft understanding of how to replace common inflammatory agents with alternatives that not only mimic their function and taste but also contribute to your overarching goal of reducing bodily inflammation.

Healthy Swaps

Learning how to implement effective ingredient swaps allows you to meticulously execute an anti-inflammatory diet without any sense of deprivation or any loss of flavor. Foundational elements like flour present a challenge when its gluten content poses a risk for inflammation in susceptible individuals. Here, almond and coconut flours emerge as viable alternatives; their rich textures and subtle flavors provide an ideal base for a range of culinary exploits, from baking to thickening sauces. Similarly, the ubiquitous presence of omega-6-rich vegetable oils in cooking calls for careful reconsideration. Olive oil offers a heart-healthy alternative for baking, roasting, and salad dressings. For higher-heat cooking, the stable and nutrient-dense avocado oil ensures the preservation of the integrity of the dish.

Gluten-Free and Dairy-Free Options

As dairy is a common provocateur of inflammatory responses, reimagining its role in recipes is warranted. Nut milks' mild flavors and creamy consistencies provide a lactose-free alternative for everything from smoothies to creamy sauces. Nutritional yeast—with its savory, cheese-like flavor and rich vitamin B content—can likewise become a staple for those seeking the umami depth of cheese without the dairy.

For gluten, the path to substitution is paved with a variety of grains and flours that cater to sensitivities without sacrificing the pleasures of baked goods and pastas. Although not true grains per se, quinoa and buckwheat offer alternatives for everything from morning porridges to hearty dinner bowls. Moreover, when used in baking, rice and oat flours can replicate the textures and flavors of their gluten-containing counterparts.

Natural Sweeteners

As sugar is a known contributor to inflammatory processes, natural sweeteners stand as beacons of hope when adjusting our diets. Honey and maple syrup, in their unrefined forms, offer more than just sweetness; they imbue dishes with complex flavors and a host of minerals and antioxidants. Their use, however, calls for moderation, as their caloric content mirrors that of sugar. Stevia and monk fruit—with their natural origins and negligible calorie content—present alternatives for those seeking sweetness without glycemic impact, and they can be used to sweeten everything from beverages to baked goods.

Creative Cooking

What primarily might feel like an obligation is in fact an invitation for creativity in the kitchen. By challenging yourself to not merely replicate traditional dishes but reinvent them, a vast palette of nature's ingredients is within reach. Guided by the principles of anti-inflammatory eating, you'll embark on an adventure leading to new, delightful yet healthy flavors, textures, and combinations.

In this endeavor, the creation of your own spice blends—using anti-inflammatory herbs and spices—adds depth and complexity to dishes, transforming simple meals into culinary delights.

From sauerkraut to kimchi, the use of fermented foods can also introduce not just unique flavors but also probiotics—allies in the maintenance of gut health and inflammation reduction. Each vegetable and fruit has its own anti-inflammatory profile, ensuring that every meal is a mosaic of nutrients that celebrates the diversity that defines both our planet and the path to health.

As you dive into an anti-inflammatory diet, your kitchen can become a place of discovery and healing. Through this lens, the challenges posed by the need for substitutions transform into opportunities to expand your culinary horizons and enrich your diet in ways that nurture both body and soul. In this journey, the ultimate reward lies not in the replication of traditional flavors but in the creation of new traditions that honor the principles of anti-inflammatory eating and celebrate the joy of discovery at the heart of culinary exploration.

Seasonal Eating: Maximizing Nutrients and Flavor

Aligning your diet with the rhythm of the seasons offers a pathway to enhance the nutritional quality and taste of your meals while fostering a deeper connection with the natural world. This alignment with the cyclical bounty of the earth not only enriches the culinary experience but also grounds our eating habits with a sense of place and time. The essence of seasonal eating lies in its ability to concentrate the freshest, most flavorful ingredients at the peak of their nutritional value directly from farm to table. Rooted in ancient traditions, this practice has gained renewed relevance in modern times as a counterbalance to the globalization of the food supply, which often prioritizes convenience over quality and nutrition.

Eating with the seasons offers a way to sustain one's health while supporting the health of the planet. The nutrient density of produce harvested at its peak is unparalleled; vitamins, minerals, and antioxidants are more available in naturally ripened produce, therefore ensuring that each bite delivers a potent dose of health-promoting compounds. Additionally, minimizing your use of out-of-season produce that requires long-distance transportation also allows you to avoid preservatives that can prompt inflammatory responses.

Furthermore, the flavors of seasonal foods are incomparable; whether it's spring's tender greens, summer's succulent fruits, autumn's hearty root vegetables, or winter's sturdy squashes, each season presents an opportunity to rediscover the joy of cooking and eating.

The benefits of this practice extend beyond the individual to the community and environment at large. By choosing seasonal, locally grown produce, you can play a vital role in sustaining local agriculture by reducing the carbon footprint associated with long-distance food transport and minimizing the reliance on preservatives and packaging needed for extended shelf life. This support bolsters the local economy, fosters a sense of community, and promotes a food system that's more resilient and sustainable. The act of purchasing local produce is a way to invest in a future of food that is both nourishing and sustainable.

Adapting your diet to the ebb and flow of the seasons requires both knowledge and flexibility. Seasonal food guides are often available from local agricultural extension services or farmers' markets, and they can be invaluable resources in this endeavor, as they offer insights into the produce that's currently at its peak. The joy of seasonal eating lies in the anticipation and discovery of each season's offerings while encouraging a diet that is diverse and rich in a broad spectrum of nutrients.

Incorporating seasonal foods into your daily meals invites innovation and experimentation. Salads become a canvas for the freshest greens, herbs, and edible flowers of spring, while summer's abundance can be captured in light, fruit-based desserts or grilled vegetable platters. Autumn calls for the warmth of soups and stews brimming with root vegetables and beans, whereas winter's harvest lends itself to roasted dishes and hearty casseroles. This approach can not only elevate your dining experience but also ensure that your diet remains dynamic and engaging, helping you to avoid impulsive decisions rooted in gustatory boredom.

Rooting your diet in the rhythms of the natural world offers a way to nourish your body with the highest quality ingredients, support the local community and economy, and tread lightly on the earth. This serves as a reminder that the impact of our dining table choices starts with our health but reflects on the planet.

In the next chapter, we'll shift our focus to the broader implications of these choices and explore how the principles of an anti-inflammatory diet intersect with the global challenges of sustainability and food security.

Chapter 4:

Dawn Delights—A Guide to Anti-Inflammatory Breakfasts

The morning sun heralds not just a new day but also a new opportunity to nourish our bodies in alignment with nature's rhythms and the wisdom of scientific research on inflammation. The breaking of the night's fast with foods that combat inflammation sets the tone of a symphony that contributes to the harmony of our health throughout the day. This chapter introduces quick and easy breakfasts as not just meals but also medicinal agents capable of influencing your body's inflammatory response from the very start of the day.

Quick and Easy Smoothies and Breakfast Bowls

Nutrient-Dense Ingredients

When considering anti-inflammatory foods, variety and nutrient density weave together to form a protective dietary strategy against inflammation. The versatility and simplicity of smoothies and breakfast bowls offer an excellent canvas for incorporating a wide range of fruits, vegetables, nuts, and seeds. Each ingredient plays a role, contributing to the overall anti-inflammatory effect. For instance, dark leafy greens such as spinach and kale can be included to enrich your body with iron and calcium, while berries can help neutralize free radicals with their high antioxidant content. Also, nuts and seeds bring omega-3 fatty acids to the table, directly combating inflammation.

Protein and Fiber

Satiety and lasting energy are the foundational stones upon which a productive day is built. Including protein and fiber in your breakfasts ensures that your energy levels remain stable, warding off mid-morning hunger pangs and the consequent reach for inflammatory snack foods. A smoothie or breakfast bowl that combines plant-based protein powder or Greek yogurt with fibrous fruits and vegetables creates a meal that is both filling and anti-inflammatory. The inclusion of a protein source is crucial for muscle repair and growth, while fiber supports digestive health and keeps blood sugar levels in check.

I personally love to make overnight oats, which we will discuss in more detail below. They are an easy grab-and-go all-in-one breakfast bowl option that offers plenty of opportunity for variety and the inclusion of both protein and fiber. My current favorite version includes lemon-flavored skyr—an Icelandic high-protein alternative to yogurt—and blueberries.

On the weekends, I favor a scrambled egg-based breakfast bowl topped with my current favorite veggies and beans or seeds—right now, I'm loving some garlic-sauteéd spinach, pico de gallo, and crushed pistachios, all of which I prep in advance to make breakfast as seamless as possible. Work with the flavors you already know you enjoy, and tweak them to create nutritionally well-rounded breakfast options. My overnight oats recipe, for instance, was inspired by my favorite flavor of cheesecake—talk about a healthier way to satisfy my cravings!

Superfood Additions

The term "superfood" might evoke images of rare and exotic ingredients that necessitate super-specific cooking methods, but in reality, these are simply foods that are rich in accessible and highly effective nutrients and antioxidants. Spirulina, chlorella, and maca powder are examples of superfoods that can be easily incorporated into smoothies and breakfast bowls for an extra anti-inflammatory boost. Spirulina is a type of blue-green algae that is lauded for its high protein content, excellently available iron, and superb anti-inflammatory properties. Chlorella also aids in detoxifying the body. Maca powder is derived from a root vegetable that is known for its energy-boosting properties and ability to balance hormones, thus indirectly supporting the body's inflammatory response. A teaspoon or two of any of these ingredients can take your smoothies and breakfast bowls to the next level.

Recipe Ideas

Crafting a nutritious, anti-inflammatory breakfast that aligns with your taste preferences and dietary needs doesn't require culinary expertise. A simple recipe might include a smoothie made with almond milk, a handful of frozen mixed berries, a scoop of plant-based protein powder, a tablespoon of flaxseeds, and a teaspoon of spirulina. For those preferring a bowl, blending frozen bananas and oats with a splash of plant-based milk creates a creamy fiber-rich base to which various toppings like nuts, seeds, and fresh fruit can be added. The key is in the combination of ingredients; each should be selected for its flavor and health benefits to create a meal that delights your senses while nourishing your body. Take a few moments now to ponder what flavor and nutrient combinations you might like to include in your next meal plan.

Visual Element: Anti-Inflammatory Smoothie Bowl Infographic

Creating an infographic of your smoothie options and preferences can visually guide you through the process of creating a balanced, nutritious breakfast bowl when you are still in a sleepy haze in the mornings. Categorize your commonly available ingredients as follows to create an easy-to-use template to smooth your morning decision-making:

- bases like avocado, banana, and yogurts

- proteins such as seeds, nuts, high-protein yogurts, and protein powders

- fruits and vegetables, particularly those that are high in essential micronutrients like berries, spinach, and kale

- superfood add-ons, including spirulina, chlorella, and maca powder

This offers a mix-and-match approach that encourages you to customize your daily breakfasts and avoid dietary stagnation.

Starting the day with a meal that fights inflammation also sets a precedent for health-conscious choices throughout the day. Smoothies and breakfast bowls—with their versatility and ease of preparation—present an ideal opportunity to incorporate a variety of anti-inflammatory foods into your diet from the very beginning of your day. With each sip or spoonful, we pledge to honor our bodies with foods that heal and energize.

Overnight Oats Variations: Prep in Your Sleep

As the world slumbers, a simple yet profound transformation can occur within the confines of our kitchens; the unassuming raw state of oats undergoes a metamorphosis and emerges at dawn as a nourishing concoction, ready to fuel the day's endeavors. This section covers overnight oats, a breakfast option that marries the simplicity of preparation with the richness of nutrition and a myriad of tastes. As I mentioned above, these are some of my favorite weekday breakfast options as they are so easy to prepare and alter to any preferences.

Base Recipe

The foundation of any overnight oats is deceptively simple, requiring nothing more than oats and a liquid, such as almond milk, left to intermingle overnight. Typically, a ratio of one part oats to two parts liquid is used, and this serves as a canvas upon which flavors and textures can be layered. The beauty of this preparation lies in its passive nature; while we surrender to sleep, the oats soften, absorbing the liquid and flavors and transforming into a creamy, ready-to-eat breakfast by morning.

Flavor Variations

Introducing a variety of flavors maintains the allure of overnight oats as a staple breakfast option. Variation not only combats the monotony of repetition but also allows for a personalized breakfast experience each morning. Tropical variations might infuse the oats with coconut milk, mango, and a squeeze of lime. Berry themes could blend mixed berries, a dollop of yogurt, and a drizzle of honey for a sweet, antioxidant-rich start to the day. Chocolate variations are indulgent yet healthful, and they might incorporate cocoa powder, a hint of vanilla, and banana slices, adding natural sweetness. Nut butter themes also offer a rich, satisfying option with a swirl of almond or peanut butter and slices of apple for crunch. Each variation, while distinct in flavor, remains anchored to the base recipe, therefore illustrating the versatility and adaptability of overnight oats as a breakfast choice. So, work with flavors that you already know you enjoy to ensure that this remains an appealing choice no matter the circumstances of your morning.

Nutritional Enhancements

Beyond flavor, the inclusion of ingredients that amplify the nutritional value of overnight oats ensures that this meal not only satisfies your hunger but also combats inflammation. When ground to ensure bioavailability, flaxseeds bring a wealth of omega-3 fatty acids essential for reducing inflammation. Chia seeds are tiny yet powerful, offering not just omega-3s but also an impressive fiber content thus aiding digestive health. Hemp hearts contribute a complete protein encompassing all essential amino acids—a rarity in plant-based ingredients. These enhancements can be stirred into the base mixture before the overnight soak to imbue the oats with a depth of nutrition that transforms them into a powerhouse of anti-inflammatory benefits.

Gluten-Free Options

For those navigating the complexities of gluten intolerance, overnight oats offer a sanctuary of flexibility. Though oats are naturally gluten-free, they are often processed in factories that could harbor the risk of cross-contamination. By selecting certified gluten-free oats, the meal remains safe and enjoyable for everyone. In the case of avenin sensitivity—an intolerance to a gluten-like substance that is present in all oats—alternative grains, such as quinoa flakes or buckwheat groats, provide a novel texture and flavor profile while maintaining the integrity of the overnight oat concept. Soaking them in a similar fashion to traditional oats expands the horizon of possibilities and ensures that the benefits of this convenient, nutritious breakfast are accessible to all, regardless of dietary restrictions.

The simplicity and depth of nutrition of this breakfast option offer a reminder that nourishment extends beyond the mere act of eating. With each variation and nutritional enhancement, overnight oats offer a simple path to healthful eating and assist us throughout the complexities of our days.

Anti-Inflammatory Breakfast Wraps and Sandwiches

When thoughtfully constructed with whole grains or gluten-free alternatives, lean proteins, an array of vegetables, and healthy fats, these handheld delights transform into bastions of anti-inflammatory goodness that are capable of fueling your body while quelling the fires of inflammation.

Whole Grain and Gluten-Free Wraps

The base of any wrap or sandwich speaks volumes of its nutritional intent. With their rich fiber content, whole grain options can be champions of gut health, as their complex carbohydrates release energy steadily, preventing the spikes in blood sugar that can provoke inflammatory responses.

For those navigating the challenges of gluten sensitivity, the market offers a plethora of alternatives, from wraps fashioned from teff or buckwheat to breads that utilize almond or coconut flour as their base. These gluten-free options also contribute their own unique textures and flavors, enhancing the eating experience while ensuring it remains inflammation-friendly.

Protein Choices

Protein is the building block of muscles and tissues, and it assumes a critical role in the construction of breakfast wraps and sandwiches. Lean animal proteins, such as eggs, offer a complete amino acid profile, each with their own additional micronutrient profiles. For example, smoked salmon is rich in omega-3 fatty acids and can be included to reflect your commitment to combating inflammation through your diet. Equally compelling are plant-based proteins like tofu and tempeh, which not only provide a high-quality protein source but also introduce phytochemicals and fiber, further contributing to the anti-inflammatory properties of the meal. The inclusion of these proteins transforms the wrap or sandwich from mere convenience food into a meal that supports bodily functions and combats inflammation at a cellular level.

Vegetable Fillings

Vegetables' vibrant diversity offers a kaleidoscope of nutrients, antioxidants, and fiber, contributing to the body's anti-inflammatory defenses. The incorporation of leafy greens, such as spinach, provides a wealth of vitamins A, C, and K, along with folate—essential nutrients that support immune function and cellular repair. Lycopene-rich tomatoes and heart-healthy avocados can further enrich your breakfast options, adding depth to their flavors as well as a multitude of health benefits. The artful integration of vegetables into your wraps and sandwiches ensures that each bite delivers a spectrum of nutrients, therefore enhancing your body's resilience against inflammation and disease.

Healthy Fats

The role of healthy fats in reducing inflammation cannot be overstated. The creamy texture and rich nutritional content of the monounsaturated fats in avocados allow them to serve as a dual-purpose ingredient. Also, the subtle sweetness of nut butters offers a satisfying richness that can complement the other flavors within a wrap or sandwich. These fats aren't just sources of energy; they're integral to the absorption of fat-soluble vitamins, the maintenance of cell membranes, and the production of anti-inflammatory compounds.

The flexibility inherent in the concept of wraps and sandwiches invites personalization, allowing you to tailor your breakfasts to meet your nutritional needs, taste preferences, and dietary restrictions. When coupled with a focus on anti-inflammatory ingredients, this adaptability positions these breakfast options as powerful tools in the maintenance of health and well-being, thus offering a delicious, practical approach to starting the day on a note of intentional nourishment.

Power-Packed Pancakes and Waffles

When we consider breakfast, the thought of pancakes and waffles often evokes memories of leisurely mornings and the comfort of home. Yet, beneath this nostalgia and their golden exterior lies an opportunity to redefine these classics as bastions of nutrition by transforming them from simple carbohydrates into vessels of anti-inflammatory prowess. Through the judicious selection of alternative flours, the infusion of nutrient-rich add-ins, strategic topping with anti-inflammatory ingredients, and enhancement with protein sources, pancakes and waffles ascend from a weekend indulgence to a weekday staple.

Alternative Flours

Traditional white flour is often linked to inflammation due to its high glycemic index and lack of nutrients. Instead, you can revolutionize your breakfast with almond, oat, and coconut flours, which have not only a gluten-free pedigree but also an impressive array of nutrients. Almond flour is rich in vitamin E and magnesium, and it offers a moist, tender texture to pancakes and waffles, along with a subtle nutty flavor that complements a variety of add-ins. Oat flour is heralded for its soluble fiber content, and it lends a heartiness to the batter that satisfies hunger and stabilizes blood sugar levels. The absorbency and density of coconut flour requires an adjustment in liquid ratios but results in a surprisingly light finish with a slight sweetness and boost of fiber. These flours' palette of diversity offers delicious yet deeply nourishing breakfasts.

Add-Ins for Nutrition

The ability to create pancakes and waffles that heal as well as delight lies in the art of ingredient incorporation. Mashed bananas reduce the need for added sugars while contributing potassium and vitamin C. Pumpkin puree—a harbinger of autumn—enriches the batter with fiber, vitamin A, and beta-carotene, and its earthy sweetness pairs well with spices like cinnamon and nutmeg. Interestingly, grated zucchini vanishes within the batter leaving behind moisture, a subtle vegetal note, and a host of nutrients including vitamin C and manganese. When carefully folded into the batter, these add-ins can transform your pancakes and waffles into meals that deliver a spectrum of anti-inflammatory nutrients.

Topping Ideas

The crowning of pancakes and waffles is traditionally a sugary affair, but it can be reimagined as an opportunity to further bolster the body's anti-inflammatory defenses. Fresh berries add a burst of color and a tangy sweetness that negates the need for excessive syrup. Nuts and seeds introduce texture, healthy fats, and a range of nutrients including omega-3 fatty acids and zinc. A drizzle of pure maple syrup or honey, used sparingly, imparts sweetness while also providing minerals and antioxidants. The careful application of these toppings not only enhances the sensory experience of breakfast but also contributes functional nutrients that support your body's fight against inflammation. My personal favorite is to top oat-and-banana pancakes with smooth peanut butter and strawberries; it's a delicious and super-filling meal that feels like a luxury despite being very simple to prepare.

Protein Boost

In the quest for a balanced breakfast that sustains your energy levels through the morning, protein is a critical component. The incorporation of egg whites into the batter increases protein content without adding excess fat resulting in fluffy, airy pancakes and waffles. Protein powders—particularly those derived from plants such as peas or brown rice—can be seamlessly integrated into the batter, bolstering the protein content while remaining unobtrusive in flavor.

Greek yogurt is an excellent base for waffle batter or a nutritious topping for pancakes, providing probiotics alongside protein. These enhancements can be strategically woven into the fabric of the recipe to ensure that your pancakes and waffles fulfill their potential as meals that balance macronutrients, consequently supporting muscle repair, growth, and overall satiety.

In this new dawn of breakfast cuisine, pancakes and waffles are not merely comfort foods but champions of nutrition and taste. The infusion of nutrient-rich add-ins transforms each dish into a mosaic of vitamins and minerals. Using nutritional toppings further turns each serving into a canvas of anti-inflammatory artistry.

You can also enhance your pancakes and waffles with protein sources to ensure that satisfaction lasts well beyond the final bite. In this reimagined form, pancakes and waffles become meals that nourish, energize, and delight, therefore proving that the first meal of the day can indeed be the most beneficial.

Savory Breakfast Ideas for Egg Lovers

When aiming for culinary versatility, eggs should be lauded for their capacity to effortlessly transition from the cornerstone of a simple meal to the stars of sophisticated dishes that delight the palate and nourish the body. This section explores the myriad ways in which eggs can be transformed into savory breakfast dishes; each variation is a testament to their indispensable place in a diet focused on mitigating inflammation.

Egg-Based Dishes

Eggs, in their simplicity, harbor the potential for remarkable culinary diversity. Omelets, for instance, provide an opportunity to encase a variety of anti-inflammatory ingredients within their tender folds. Frittatas, with their hearty depth and rustic appeal, allow for the incorporation of leftovers, ensuring that no nutrient-rich vegetable is wasted as a result. Shakshuka—a dish steeped in tradition and bursting with taste—bathes eggs in a spicy tomato and pepper sauce thus imbuing them with a richness that belies the simplicity of its preparation. Each dish underlines the adaptability of eggs, making them an invaluable ally in the quest for an anti-inflammatory yet alluring breakfast.

Vegetable Integration

The infusion of vegetables into egg-based dishes elevates them from mere protein sources to comprehensive meals that offer a spectrum of anti-inflammatory benefits. Spinach, wilted just slightly within an omelet, contributes iron and calcium alongside its subtle bitterness, while mushrooms, sautéed until golden, add a meaty texture along with selenium, a powerful antioxidant. Whether sweet or fiery, peppers can introduce vitamin C and capsaicin, consequently enhancing the dish's flavor profile and its anti-inflammatory prowess. A deliberate integration of vegetables can transform your breakfast plate into a vibrant tableau of health-promoting ingredients.

Healthy Cooking Methods

The method by which eggs and their accompaniments are cooked significantly impacts their nutritional value and their role in an anti-inflammatory diet. Poaching is a technique that envelops the egg in a gentle bath of water, and it preserves its delicate structure and nutrients while offering a textural contrast that's both pleasing to the palate and beneficial to the body. Baking—particularly in the case of frittatas—allows for the slow melding of flavors with minimal need for added fats, therefore ensuring that the dish remains light yet satisfying. Light sautéing—preferably in a small amount of avocado oil—ensures that vegetables retain their crunch and nutrient density. Careful selection of your cooking methods, with an eye toward preserving and enhancing the nutritional content of the ingredients, ensures that your breakfast plate is as healthful as it is delicious.

Herbs and Spices

No exploration of egg-based dishes would be complete without a nod to the transformative power of herbs and spices—nature's own medicine cabinet. With its vibrant hue and potent anti-inflammatory compound (curcumin), turmeric infuses dishes with a warmth that is both culinary and medicinal. Garlic can be minced and sautéed until fragrant, and it offers allicin, known for its immune-boosting properties. From the verdant brightness of parsley to the aromatic depths of rosemary and thyme, fresh herbs not only elevate the flavor profile of an egg-based dish but also contribute a range of phytochemicals that support the body's anti-inflammatory mechanisms. The judicious use of these healthy yet tasty seasonings ensures that each egg-based breakfast is a step toward wellness.

In the realm of savory breakfasts, eggs are unrivaled in their capacity to unify a diverse array of ingredients into cohesive dishes that are both nurturing and immensely satisfying. Their versatility invites a creative exploration of flavors, textures, and nutrients that align with the principles of an anti-inflammatory diet. Through the incorporation of the elements above, eggs transcend their humble origins to become the cornerstone of anti-inflammatory breakfasts to effectively kick-start your day and also support your body's natural defenses against inflammation. This journey through the possibilities inherent in egg-based dishes serves as a reminder of the joy and health that can be found in the simple yet daily ritual of cooking and eating.

Gluten-Free Morning Pastries: Scones, Muffins, and More

To intertwine health with indulgence, gluten-free morning pastries exemplify the creativity and adaptability at the heart of anti-inflammatory cooking. In gluten-free baking, the conventional is reimagined, giving rise to scones, muffins, and quick breads that delight the palate while adhering to anti-inflammatory principles.

Gluten-Free Baking Tips

While initially daunting, the transition to gluten-free baking unveils possibilities where the limitations imposed by traditional wheat flour dissolve. The mastery over a blend of flours that mimic the structure and texture of wheat flour is key. When balanced correctly, a mix combining rice and tapioca flours—for their mild flavor and chewy texture—with almond flour, for richness and moisture, creates a base that rivals its gluten-containing counterpart. The addition of xanthan gum—a binder that is commonly used in the absence of gluten—ensures that the dough or batter retains its cohesion, therefore preventing the crumbly outcome often associated with gluten-free baked goods. When paired with an understanding of each flour's unique properties, this foundational knowledge sets the stage for successful gluten-free baking.

Nutrient-Dense Ingredients

The essence of anti-inflammatory baking lies not just in the removal of gluten but in the incorporation of ingredients that elevate the nutritional profile of the pastries. More than a wheat flour alternative, almond flour enriches baked goods with protein, fiber, and vitamin E—a potent antioxidant. When used as a partial substitute for flour or as an egg replacement, flaxseeds introduce omega-3 fatty acids, known for their anti-inflammatory effects. Pureed fruits, such as applesauce or pumpkin, offer natural sweetness, therefore reducing the need for added sugars while imbuing the pastries with vitamins and moisture. The intentional selection and use of nutrient-dense ingredients ensures that each pastry not only satisfies your craving for something sweet and comforting but also contributes to your body's nutritional needs. I love to add pumpkin seeds and sunflower seeds to my gluten-free savory scones as an additional hit of flavor, texture, protein, and omega-3s.

Healthy Swaps

Inherent in the philosophy of anti-inflammatory baking is the principle of substitution, where traditional pastry ingredients that may exacerbate inflammation are replaced with healthier alternatives. The natural sweetness and moisture of applesauce can step in for oil and butter, reducing the saturated fat content while maintaining a tender crumb. With glycemic impacts moderated by their antioxidant content, maple syrup and honey can offer a depth of flavor that replaces traditional sugars. Also, dark chocolate with a high cocoa content minimizes sugar intake while indulging the senses. These swaps are subtle yet impactful, and they redefine morning pastries as allies in the quest for health without compromising on taste or enjoyment.

Recipe Ideas

The culmination of this exploration into gluten-free, anti-inflammatory baking is a collection of suggested dishes that can act as a beacon for those seeking to start their day with something sweet yet beneficial. Scones' golden crusts and soft interiors can feature flavors from blueberry and lemon to savory cheddar and chive. Muffins can be studded with nuts, seeds, or dark chocolate chips to become portable morning meals, dense with nutrients and flavor. Next, quick breads—spanning from banana walnut to zucchini—offer slices of comfort that are embedded with the richness that gluten-free baking can achieve. This collection stands as proof of the joy and satisfaction that can be found in pastries crafted with health in mind.

Gluten-free pastries are laden with comfort and nostalgia, and they can be more than mere alternatives but rather preferred choices. Through the implementation of the strategies above, these baked goods can be a key element of a diet that values both health and pleasure.

The breakfast ideas offered in this chapter remind us that eating well doesn't necessitate sacrifice but invites creativity and a daily opportunity to nourish our bodies while delighting our senses. As we move forward, let this exploration serve as a guide, illuminating the path toward a diet that embraces the principles of anti-inflammatory eating.

Chapter 5:

Midday Morsels—Nourishing the

Noon

When the sun claims the sky and the morning's energy begins to wane, the call for noon nourishment rings clear. The choices made at lunch can either amplify or unravel the morning's good work and, thus, set the stage for vitality or fatigue as the day unfolds. From this perspective, crafting satisfying yet nourishing meals becomes an act of self-care.

Within this framework, salads emerge not as mere sides but as centerpieces—vibrant and delicious delights made up of the freshest produce, lean proteins, and whole grains. They stand as proof that food can be both medicine and pleasure—a dual role that speaks to both our bodies' needs and our palates' desires.

Salads That Satisfy: Beyond the Greens

Protein-Rich Additions

The addition of protein to a salad transforms it from a simple appetizer to a substantial meal capable of fueling your body through the afternoon slump. Picture a bustling farmer's market on a sunny morning, stalls brimming with the season's bounty: You'll find the ingredients for your next meal among the vibrant hues of fresh produce. Grilled chicken lends its smoky depth to the crispness of the greens. Tofu can be marinated in a mix of soy sauce, garlic, and ginger to offer a plant-based alternative that is both hearty and flavorful. Beans—whether black, kidney, or garbanzo—add a creamy texture and a boost of fiber.

Whole Grains

The integration of whole grains into salads introduces not just texture and substance but a host of nutritional benefits. Quinoa's subtle nuttiness, farro's chewy resilience, and brown rice's comforting familiarity show us the diversity and versatility of grains. These grains act as a sponge, absorbing the flavors of the dressing and thus consolidating a cohesive whole.

Homemade Dressings

Homemade dressings can elevate a salad from the mundane to the sublime. With olive oil as the base, additional lemon zest and juice or vinegar introduce a bright acidity that balances the oil's richness. Freshly chopped herbs lend their aromatic notes, while a touch of honey or maple syrup adds a subtle sweetness that rounds out the flavors. Whisked together in your kitchen, this concoction can become more than just a dressing; it's a declaration of intent—a commitment to nourishing your body with every drop.

Creative Combinations

The art of salad composition lies in the balance of flavors, textures, and colors. Consider this roasted vegetable salad: caramelized edges of parsnips and carrots mingled with the smoky char of bell peppers, all atop a bed of arugula dressed in a balsamic vinaigrette. Or you might prefer a grain salad in which quinoa serves as the backdrop for a medley of cucumbers, tomatoes, and feta. Asian-inspired slaw—a crunchy riot of colors from red cabbage, carrots, and green onions dressed in a peanut-ginger sauce—offers a playful twist on tradition. The endless possibilities that salads offer invite you to explore new flavors and textures within the framework of anti-inflammatory eating.

Visual Element: Salad Composition Chart

As with other dishes that can offer a near-overwhelming level of variety, it can be hugely helpful to put together a chart titled, *The Anatomy of a Satisfying Salad*. Here, you can break down the components of a salad into categories: leafy greens, protein sources, whole grains, vegetables and fruits, extras (nuts, seeds, cheeses), and dressings. Each category should include a variety of options with icons representing each item. This will streamline your decision-making process when composing a salad and empower you to mix and match components based on your personal preferences and nutritional goals. This tool can serve as a guide for constructing nourishing and fulfilling salads and a visual reminder of their diversity and flexibility in the pursuit of health.

Soups and Stews: Comfort in a Bowl

Across the culinary traditions that span the globe, soups and stews hold a revered place by offering solace and sustenance with each spoonful. These dishes serve as vessels for the nourishing embrace of the earth's bounty. The creation of soups and stews that align with anti-inflammatory principles adds an additional layer of intention to this culinary practice.

Broth-Based Options

The foundation of any noteworthy soup or stew is its broth— water imbued with the essence of herbs, vegetables, and sometimes, proteins. Vegetable broth offers a mineral-rich base teeming with phytonutrients. Chicken broth—slow-simmered to extract collagen, amino acids, and minerals from bones—provides a comforting depth, while beef bone broth is famous for its healing properties and acts as a potent elixir for gut health and inflammation reduction. Simmered over low heat, these broths become repositories of both flavor and nutrition. When you don't have the time, energy, or inclination to create your own broths, look for bouillon options at your local grocery store to get the most flavor and nutrition from prepackaged options.

Legume-Laden Recipes

The incorporation of legumes into soups and stews stands as a testament to their versatility and nutritional prowess. Red lentils dissolve into a velvety consistency in soups, acting as both a thickening agent and a powerful source of nutrition as their fiber and protein content support digestive health and satiety. When stewed with spices and vegetables, black beans offer a robust base for hearty stews, and their anthocyanins and fiber work in concert to modulate inflammation. The humble garbanzo bean, when simmered, becomes a creamy beacon of plant-based protein and iron. These legumes are ancient staples of diets around the world, and they not only extend the heartiness of soups and stews but also their healing potential, offering a confluence of nutrients essential for combating inflammation.

Vegetable-Forward Choices

As we have discussed, vegetables are a vital element of any anti-inflammatory diet. Soups and stews that prioritize vegetables invite a celebration of the seasons, with each spoonful a reflection of the land's current nutritional offerings. A summer soup might sing with the brightness of tomatoes and zucchini, their lycopene and saponins mingling in a light broth. Autumn stews can lean into the earthiness of root vegetables, their beta-carotene and antioxidants seeping into the rich liquid. This focus on vegetables not only elevates the nutritional profile of soups and stews but also their aesthetic appeal.

Slow-Cooker and Instant-Pot Methods

The modern kitchen boasts tools that simplify the process of soup and stew making by intertwining convenience with culinary tradition. Slow cookers offer a promise of "set and forget," gently coaxing flavors from ingredients over hours. Instant Pots—also known as pressure cookers—on the other hand, are champions of efficiency, as they reduce cooking times in their pressurized environment without sacrificing flavor or nutrition. These emblems of contemporary cooking allow you to craft dishes that respect the hustle of daily life while honoring your body's need for nourishing and healing meals. The adaptation of recipes to these appliances—whether it be a bone broth simmered overnight in a slow cooker or a lentil stew brought to life in an Instant Pot—reflects your commitment to feeding your body well amidst the whirlwind of modern existence.

When guided by the principles of anti-inflammatory eating, eating soups and stews transcends into an act of healing. The broths that serve as the foundation, the legumes that impart heartiness, the vegetables that offer their nutrients freely, and the methods that marry convenience with tradition all converge in dishes that comfort the body as much as they soothe the soul.

Hearty Wraps and Sandwiches With a Twist

We have already touched on the powerful variety of breakfast wraps and sandwiches, but when it comes to lunches, these convenient options emerge as a culinary refuge—a moment stolen from the day's demands. Hand-held meals find new expression through the lens of anti-inflammatory eating, where each ingredient is chosen not just for its taste but for its capacity to heal and energize on the go.

Innovative Wraps

Exploring the breadth of nature's bounty provides us with plenty of inspiration for how to create tantalizing alternative wraps. Collard greens, with their broad, sturdy leaves, offer a gluten-free substitute for the traditional wheat tortilla. The delicate, pure layers of crispy and refreshing lettuce leaves present a lighter option. Gluten-free tortillas, though born from the necessity of dietary restrictions, provide a bridge between tradition and innovation. This reimagining of the wrap from a mere vessel to a vibrant component of the meal underscores the philosophy of anti-inflammatory eating, where every element on the plate serves a purpose beyond satiation.

Unique Fillings

The fillings you choose can diverge from the mundane and embrace the unique and the flavorful. Caramelized and sweet roasted vegetables bring warmth and depth, their fibrous bodies rich in nutrients and antioxidants. Since creamy and earthy hummus has a base of garbanzo beans—which are a potent source of protein and fiber—it can act as both a spread and a health-promoting substance. Avocado adds a lushness to each bite, while tiny yet tenacious sprouts offer a crunch that belies their nutritional heft. This ensemble of fillings—each selected for its health benefits and flavor profile—can transform your wrap or sandwich from a quick meal into a nuanced exploration of taste and nourishment.

Balanced Combinations

An effective balance of macronutrients ensures sustained energy and satiety. Carbohydrates can be drawn from greens or gluten-free tortillas to provide the body's preferred source of fuel. Proteins—whether animal-based or derived from soy, legumes, and seeds—offer the building blocks for repair and growth; their presence ensures muscle health and metabolic balance. Fats—particularly those of the unsaturated variety found in avocados and nuts—contribute to satiety and the absorption of fat-soluble vitamins, rounding out the meal with a sense of completeness and well-being. When coupled with the micro-nutrients and phytochemicals in the vegetables and spices, this strategic blend of macronutrients creates a meal that's not just filling but fundamentally nourishing—a midday reprieve that can reinvigorate your body and mind.

Sauce and Spread Options

To these carefully constructed bases and fillings, sauces and spreads add the final flourish—a moistening element that binds the components while infusing the meal with flavor and additional nutrients. Pesto's base of basil and pine nuts brings a vibrant green punch of antioxidants alongside its anti-inflammatory olive oil base. Tzatziki offers a cool and tangy probiotic boost with its cucumber and dill imbuing the wrap or sandwich with freshness and zest. Guacamole is a crowd favorite, and it combines the creamy richness of avocado with the sharpness of onion and the brightness of lime, creating a spread that's as beneficial to health as it's delightful to the palate. These easy and versatile sauces and spreads not only enhance the taste and texture of the meal but also contribute to its anti-inflammatory profile.

From these examples, you can clearly see that the choice of innovative wraps extends the possibilities of the meal by offering a base that is both nutritious and accommodating to dietary needs. Additionally, diverse fillings provide a canvas for creativity, and an appropriate balance of macronutrients ensures that each creation is not just a pleasure to eat but a source of sustained energy, supporting the body's needs through the trials of the day. Finally, sauces and spreads can crown your lunch with a touch of indulgence—a reminder that eating well can and should be a joy. Transformed from the ordinary into the extraordinary, the humble wrap and sandwich are reborn as a midday meal that delights your senses while fortifying your body against the challenges of inflammation and the demands of life.

Quick Stir-Fries: Veggie-Packed and Flavorful

When time is of the essence and the hunger for both sustenance and vitality grows with the advancing day, a stir-fry can be your culinary hero. This cooking method wields the power to coax a symphony of tastes from the simplest ingredients, transforming a quick lunch into an opportunity to nourish your body deeply and deliberately. At their core, the stir-fries celebrate the abundance of the earth by welcoming a myriad of vegetables and proteins; each addition is a deliberate choice aimed at reducing inflammation and elevating wellness.

The essence of stir-fries lies in their inherent versatility, a characteristic that invites the use of whatever ingredients lie ready at hand. You can use any veggies that happen to be in your refrigerator—from crisp bell peppers to tender snow peas—since each harbors its own unique blend of vitamins, minerals, and antioxidants. A stir-fry combines these vegetables, along with a carefully selected protein, bringing them together in a vibrant display of culinary improvisation. This allows for the creation of meals that are as nutritionally rich as they are visually appealing, with each ingredient retaining its texture and nutrient content through the quick application of heat.

Sauce selection is crucial when preparing a stir-fry. Homemade sauces, without added sugars and processed additives, stand as pillars of healthful cooking. You can use coconut aminos—a soy sauce alternative that is lower in sodium and devoid of soy—as the base; its savory sweetness can be enhanced by the warmth of fresh ginger, minced to release its pungent essence. Finely chopped garlic joins the chorus against inflammation. A splash of rice vinegar adds a balancing acidity, while a touch of sesame oil can be used sparingly to impart a nutty richness. Since this concoction can be whisked together in moments, it's a testament to the power of natural ingredients to elevate a dish from the mundane to the extraordinary.

Your choice of protein in a stir-fry should speak to both your preferences and nutritional strategy; the selection ranges from the lean cuts of chicken to the succulent pieces of shrimp. For those seeking plant-based alternatives, tofu (pressed to remove excess moisture) offers a blank canvas ready to absorb all flavors. The nutty texture and fermentation-derived benefits of tempeh introduce both protein and probiotics thus supporting gut health and muscle maintenance. These quick-to-cook proteins are rich in essential nutrients and can integrate seamlessly into your stir-fries while bringing their unique profile to the table.

The preparation of vegetables and proteins in advance provides extra opportunities for a quick and flavorful stir-fry, promising healthy meals within minutes. Vegetables should be sliced into uniform pieces to ensure even cooking, and they can await their turn in airtight containers. Proteins can be marinated, if desired, for added flavor and cut into bite-sized pieces, ready to meet the heat of the pan. This mindful assembly of ingredients ensures that the act of creating a stir-fry is not just a response to hunger but a deliberate act of self-care.

A skillet or wok is the stage upon which ingredients intertwine, and high heat is used to seal in flavors and preserve tender textures. By continually stirring atop this high heat, your vibrant and crisp vegetables will retain their nutritional integrity and perfectly cooked proteins can offer their tender richness to the dish.

When vegetables and proteins come together in a harmony of flavors under the guiding hand of homemade stir-fry sauces, your midday meal transcends its utilitarian roots; it becomes a vibrant expression of culinary creativity that reinforces wellness and prompts inflammation reduction.

Plant-Based Lunch Ideas for Everyone

The pivot toward dishes crafted entirely from plants is not merely a dietary preference but a conscious choice for health—a nod to the vast evidence supporting the anti-inflammatory benefits of eschewing animal products in favor of nature's harvest.

Plant-based recipes containing health-promoting ingredients can be a delicious path to improving your vitality: A lentil and sweet potato stew, simmered with cumin and coriander, is a comforting yet anti-inflammatory lunch option. A quinoa salad with beet and spinach and dressed in a lemon-tahini sauce sings with the flavors of the Mediterranean, proving the diet's versatility and its focus on whole, unprocessed foods.

In a plant-based diet, the cornerstone of fulfilling and refreshing lunches, protein, emerges not from the animal kingdom but from the earth's generous yield. Lentils have a near-complete amino acid profile and unparalleled fiber content, and their gentle flavor offers a canvas ready for many seasoning possibilities. From the creamy depths of hummus to the crisp edges of falafel, garbanzo beans lend themselves to a range of culinary applications. Quinoa and soy stand out for their complete protein contents—a rare trait in plant-based foods—making them invaluable additions to salads, bowls, and wraps. These sources of plant protein support the body's needs without the need for animal products.

As you consider incorporating more plant-based meals into your dietary repertoire, it's important to contemplate whether you wish to eliminate dairy—a staple in many diets yet a source of inflammation for some. Dairy-free alternatives offer a path forward—a way to enjoy the creamy richness of dairy without its potential drawbacks. Cashew cheese has a velvety texture and nutty flavor, making it a worthy substitute in sandwiches and salads. Additionally, coconut yogurt—tangy, smooth, and gut-healthy—serves as an excellent base for dressings and dips. These alternatives and more can turn limitations into opportunities for creativity and discovery while reflecting the diet's ethos.

A midday plant-based meal speaks to the possibility of satisfaction without sacrifice. Through the careful selection of ingredients, artful combination of textures and flavors, and thoughtful incorporation of protein and dairy alternatives, plant-based lunches remind us that food, in its most fundamental form, is a gift from the earth.

Lunchbox Snacks: Healthy On-the-Go Options

Our midday pauses for nourishment so often occur away from the sanctity of home or even the office breakroom, which necessitates meals that can travel with us. Within this context, deciding on your lunchbox snacks involves a meticulous selection of foods that not only journey well but also sustain, energize, and align with anti-inflammatory principles.

Primarily, portable and nonperishable snacks should bear resilience against the rigors of travel, ensuring they arrive as intended. With their compact size and dense nutritional profile, nuts and seeds stand out as paragons of portability. Almonds, walnuts, and pumpkin seeds offer not just a crunchy respite from hunger but a boost of energy and a bulwark against inflammation. Homemade granola bars combine oats, nuts, seeds, and dried fruits with the subtle sweetness of honey or maple syrup to create a snack that can satisfy your sweet tooth while providing sustained energy. These carefully packed companions can easily offer nourishment away from the kitchen.

Crisp and vibrant cut vegetables are a perfect counterpoint to the creamy richness of hummus. This simple yet profoundly satisfying pairing delivers a spectrum of nutrients from fiber to protein. Additionally, fresh fruit, when coupled with nut butter, transforms into a treat that balances sweetness with the satiating properties of healthy fats and protein—a harmonious blend that curbs hunger without spiking blood sugar.

Providing for the craving for something sweet but healthy addresses the midday longing for indulgence by offering deliberate delight rather than impulsive derailment. Recipes that harness the natural sweetness of fruits, the richness of nuts, and the wholesomeness of whole grains create snacks that rise above mere indulgence. Date and nut energy balls rolled in shredded coconut or cocoa powder are nutritional powerhouses, each bite dense with flavor and anti-inflammatory benefits. The simple yet nutritious baked apple chips sprinkled with cinnamon offer a crispy alternative to traditional snack foods.

The critical importance of hydration is often overlooked in the planning of meals, but it increases in the context of anti-inflammatory eating. The myriad of health benefits of drinks like herbal teas— ranging from digestive support to antioxidant properties—offers a soothing counterpoint to the day's stresses. Infused waters carry the subtle flavors and nutrients of fruits, herbs, and spices, and they provide a refreshing alternative to sugary beverages. We must remember that liquids are vital in maintaining balance and health, and their presence in our lunchboxes is a nod to a holistic approach to nourishment.

In the assembly of these lunchbox snacks, we should aim to respect the rhythm of the day and the body's needs as it navigates life's complexities. The selection of portable, non-perishable items ensures that wherever the day leads, nourishment is never far behind. Fresh snack ideas bring the vibrancy of nature's bounty into the midday meal; sweet but healthy treats address the innate desire for indulgence; hydration underscores the importance of balance between solid foods and fluids. Together, these snacks support our bodies' anti-inflammatory processes while catering to our palates' desire for variety and flavor.

As this chapter draws to a close, the essentials of crafting nourishing lunches stand clear: The principles of anti-inflammatory eating, far from being confined to the home, extend their reach into the broader canvas of life. This approach is meticulous in its attention to detail and broad in its embrace of variety, and it sets the stage for meals that not only satiate but also heal.

Chapter 6:

Evening Elixirs—Nurturing the Night

As daylight dims and the evening assumes its tranquil cloak, the kitchen becomes a haven—a place where the day's toils are set aside in favor of nourishment. One-pot meals are a game-changer when it comes to dinners, offering both simplicity and sustenance. This chapter delves into the heart of one-pot wonders, where nutrient-dense ingredients, spices, and herbs meld their flavors in a single pot under the slow caress of heat to produce not just meals but a balm for the soul.

Why One-Pot Wonders Can Work for You

Simplicity and Convenience

The allure of one-pot meals lies not just in their outcome but in their process. They have a streamlined cooking process wherein the preparation of ingredients, their cooking, and even the eventual cleanup coalesce into a singular, seamless flow. The ease of this process means that the act of creating a one-pot meal can even become a moment for mindful meditation—a deliberate slowing down where each step, from the chopping of vegetables to the gentle stirring of the pot, becomes a moment of mindfulness. The result is a meal that transcends the sum of its parts, creating a dish that's rich in flavors and textures.

Nutrient-Dense Ingredients

The ease of cooking one-pot meals allows more mental energy to be spent on the selection of ingredients that offer both flavor and anti-inflammatory nutrition. Consider the humble lentil, its earthy tones a perfect complement to the vibrant hues of tomatoes and carrots, or the robustness of lean chicken simmered with kale and quinoa. Choosing what to include is a balancing act, wherein proteins, grains, and vegetables come together in a harmony that's both pleasing to the palate and nourishing to the body. An emphasis on variety ensures that a broad spectrum of vitamins, minerals, and antioxidants can transform your one-pot meals from mere convenience to vessels of health.

Herbs and Spices for Flavor

The infusion of spices and herbs into one-pot meals offers additional flavor and anti-inflammatory properties to your dinners. From the smoky depth of paprika and the bright zest of lemon to the peppery bite of basil and the earthy undertones of rosemary, each herb and spice contributes its unique profile to the dish. When used with intention, this culinary palette not only enhances the flavors of the ingredients but also introduces an array of health benefits: Turmeric brings its anti-inflammatory prowess, cinnamon its blood sugar regulating capabilities, and garlic its immune-boosting properties. The judicious use of these seasonings elevates any one-pot meal.

Examples

The preparation of a one-pot meal offers as much flavor as it does simplicity. Picture a Dutch oven, its heavy base the perfect vessel for a slow-simmered stew where tender and rich beef melds with the sweetness of onions, the tang of tomatoes, and a dash of thyme to create a dish rich in depth and complexity. Or imagine a skillet, where salmon's pink and succulent flesh cooks amidst a medley of asparagus, potatoes, and a sprinkle of dill and lemon weaving in freshness and zest. These are just two of the myriad possibilities one-pot meals offer. Feel free to experiment. Spanish paella is one of my absolute favorite one-pot options, and its saffron is a powerful antioxidant that my body is always grateful for.

In the modern world, where time is a precious commodity and the need for nourishment is paramount, one-pot meals helpfully combine simplicity and health. They represent a return to the basics of cooking, where the act of preparing a meal is as much about feeding the soul as it is about sustaining the body. Through the careful selection of ingredients, artful use of spices and herbs, and experimentation with recipes that span cultures and cuisines, you can reconnect with the joy of cooking while packing a powerful anti-inflammatory punch with your nutrition.

Family-Friendly Dinners Everyone Will Love

For families, the preparation of dinner becomes an opportunity for unity. Therefore, it is important to craft meals that appeal to the diverse palates of both young and seasoned members of the family, while ensuring these dishes brim with nutritional merit.

Kid-Approved Recipe Ideas

The landscape of children's tastes is often a minefield of preferences and aversions, and navigating it requires a blend of culinary finesse and nutritional acumen. The secret lies in using recipes that disguise the wholesomeness of their ingredients under the cloak of familiar favorites. Envision, for instance, a pizza where the golden and inviting crust is crafted from whole grains, or even cauliflower, and its surface is lavished with a vibrant tomato sauce simmered with herbs, crowned with a medley of vegetables and a sprinkle of cheese. Also, the humble garbanzo bean can be transformed into nuggets with crisp exteriors and soft and flavorful interiors that can accompany dips that range from yogurt to beet hummus. These dishes aren't meals but gateways to a lifetime of healthy eating.

Involving the Family

Meal preparation is often consigned to be a solitary endeavor by an adult, but it holds untapped potential as a conduit for familial bonding. Inviting members, young and old, to partake in the culinary process transforms cooking from a chore to an adventure, ensuring that everyone has a stake in the meal and feels open to trying new anti-inflammatory ingredients.

It begins with the selection of recipes—a democratic process where each voice finds acknowledgment—and extends to chopping, stirring, and seasoning. Including children not only demystifies the kitchen for the younger members but also imbues them with a sense of accomplishment and belonging, with the meal as a shared victory at the day's end.

Balancing Flavors and Nutrition

At the heart of family-friendly dinners lies the delicate equilibrium between the allure of flavors and the imperative of nutrition. Achieving this balance demands a culinary strategy that introduces new foods subtly. Their richness of sweet potatoes, roasted until their sugars caramelize, offers a sweet counterpoint to the savory, and finely grated carrots can go unnoticed amidst the layers of a lasagna that uses whole grain pasta. Zucchini can be spiralized into noodles to become a playful substitute for pasta. Through repeated exposures where new ingredients aren't a challenge but a natural component of meals, the family palate will expand and embrace diversity without resistance.

Quick and Easy Options

In the ceaseless whirl of family life, time is a commodity as precious as any, and the allure of quick and easy dinner options becomes undeniable. Yet, convenience need not be the enemy of nutrition. The secret lies in leveraging the bounty of nature's fast foods—fruits, vegetables, grains, and lean proteins—in recipes that come together with grace and speed. As we discussed in the previous chapter, a stir-fry is a meal that materializes in minutes—less than the time it takes for the family to gather at the table. Soup is another excellent option; where lentils and vegetables can simmer into a wholesomeness that can be topped with coconut milk and served with whole grain bread in under 30 minutes. These meals are swift to prepare and stand as bastions of health, ensuring that even on the busiest of nights, dinner remains a sanctuary of nutrition and togetherness.

In this symphony of family dinners, the kitchen reclaims its ancient role as the heart of the home. It becomes a place where meals are not just cooked but crafted with intention, where recipes serve not merely to feed but to nurture, and where the act of eating together becomes a ritual imbued with meaning. Embark on an anti-inflammatory culinary journey through the shared adventure of cooking that celebrates the joy of eating together without compromising your health.

Date Night Dinners: Special Yet Simple

Date night dinners at home seek not just to satiate hunger but also to create an experience through the shared connection of two souls. This pursuit, while noble in its aim, need not be Herculean in its execution. In fact, the most profound experiences often stem from the humblest of origins.

Elevated Meals at Home

The boundless potential of home cooking empowers you to create dishes that whisper of elegance while avoiding complexity or inflammatory challenges. Strands of whole-grain spaghetti may entwine with the richness of olive oil, the briny kiss of capers, and the tender sweetness of cherry tomatoes, while you and your partner follow their example. A simple piece of roasted salmon with a crust of herbs and citrus zest is a delicacy that resonates with freshness, vitality, and thoughtful preparation—something that won't be left unnoticed by your other half.

Healthy Indulgences

The notion of indulgence is often shrouded in the excesses of rich sauces and decadent desserts, but it finds redefinition within the context of anti-inflammatory date night dinners. Here, indulgence is not abandonment but an embrace of ingredients that lavish the body with nutrients while delighting the palate. A dessert might take the form of poached pears bathed in a reduction of red wine and spices. Or consider the richness and depth of a dark chocolate mousse whipped into lightness with the creaminess of avocado. These dishes are indulgent yet wholesomely crafted, serving as a reminder that pleasure and health need not be mutually exclusive; they can coexist while enhancing each other.

Ambiance and Presentation

The setting in which a meal is consumed can elevate the mundane to the magical. The soft and flattering flicker of candles creates an atmosphere of intimacy. The vibrant colors and subtle fragrances of flowers add a touch of nature's beauty to the table and a visual feast that complements the culinary one. And dishes in which each element is arranged not just for ease of eating but for aesthetic pleasure transform the act of dining into an art form. A swirl of sauce here and a sprinkle of herbs there are not just an enhancement of flavor but a visual cue to the thought and care invested in the meal, and they offer an added opportunity to imbue the meal with anti-inflammatory properties. This seemingly superficial attention to ambiance and presentation enhances the dining experience and elevates it from mere sustenance to a celebration of the moment and the company while standing firm in your commitment to your well-being.

Wine Pairings

Pairing wine with food adds a layer of complexity and enjoyment to the dining experience. The selection of organic or biodynamic wines mirrors the ethos of anti-inflammatory eating. The acidity and fruitiness of a crisp, unoaked chardonnay are vibrant counterparts to the lightness of fish or poultry. Moreover, the subtle tannins and notes of red fruit in a light-bodied, biodynamic pinot noir elegantly accompany pasta dishes or a simple roast. The thoughtful pairing of wine and food serves not just to elevate the meal but to deepen the connection between you and your partner through a mutual journey through flavors and aromas.

In the creation of date night dinners, simplicity melds with elegance, indulgence with health, and ambiance with presentation. Thus, the kitchen transforms into a stage, the cook a performer, and the meal an expression of love and care.

Slow-Cooker and Instant-Pot Magic

As we discussed in the section on soups and stews in Chapter 5, the modern marvels of slow and pressure cookers are champions of convenience, and when it comes to dinners, they invite a deliberate way to ease your evening routines.

Set It and Forget It

The allure of these appliances lies in their silent pact with the cook: a promise to shoulder the day's culinary burdens. When using a slow cooker, you can layer the ingredients into the vessel during the cool clarity of morning. With the lid secured, the device is left to its task and you are freed from the tether of pots and pans with the assurance of a meal awaiting at day's end. This liberation transforms the kitchen from a place of labor to one of anticipation, where the slow melding of flavors under a device's watchful care culminates in a dinner that serves not just to satisfy hunger but to restore the spirit.

Recipes for Every Season

As the wheel of the year turns, your slow cooker and Instant Pot can adapt with grace reflecting the bounty of each season. During the winter, a root vegetable stew with tough cuts of meat can bubble gently in a slow cooker or soothing soup can be put together in minutes in a pressure cooker. Spring welcomes lighter fare where the freshness of the season's first produce shines bright against creamy grains, perhaps in an Instant-Pot chicken and asparagus risotto. Summer's abundance finds its match in a slow-cooked ratatouille—a meal that carries the scent of gardens and the promise of nutritional abundance. Finally, as autumn's chill whispers of change, a squash and bean chili—that could be cooked with either device—offers warmth with its spices as a gentle flame against the coolness. These recipes are attuned to the rhythm of the seasons, ensuring that the table remains a place of connection to the natural world, its cycles, and its gifts as well as an opportunity for nutritional variety that promotes well-being.

Maximizing Flavor

Unlocking the full potential of flavors within the confines of a slow cooker or Instant Pot demands preparation and patience. Browning meats before they surrender to the slow cooker's embrace layers the final dish with complexity. The deglazing of the pan with broth or wine—the liquid swirling into the remnants of searing—ensures that no note of flavor is lost. With an Instant Pot, the sauté function can be a beneficial prelude to pressure cooking, for instance, by releasing the fragrances of onions and garlic before adding the main ingredients. The choice of liquids—whether a homemade stock, tomato juice, or coconut milk—infuses the dish with a resonance of flavors and anti-inflammatory goodness, therefore turning the simple act of cooking into a symphony of taste and health.

Variety of Dishes

The versatility of the slow cooker and Instant Pot knows no bounds. From the clarity of a broth-based consommé to the richness of a cream-laden chowder, soups find their textures and layers of flavor enhanced by the gentle or swift processes these appliances offer. The humble ingredients of stews transform into dishes of surprising complexity—meat falling apart at a fork's touch and vegetables melding into a sauce with perfect tenderness. Roasts, which are a centerpiece of many a family meal, emerge succulent and flavorful— the meat infused with the aromatics and liquids that have been its companions in cooking. Vegetarian meals also become a testament to these devices' ability to create delicious dishes, rendering plant-based ingredients into meals that comfort and satisfy. This array of dishes showcases the adaptability of the slow cooker and Instant Pot. Regardless of your inclination or the season's offering, these appliances stand ready to transform anti-inflammatory ingredients into meals that nurture and delight.

Seafood Specialties: Light and Nourishing

Seafood, in its splendid variety, offers both delicious sources of protein and a wealth of anti-inflammatory wellness. Oily fish, in particular, glisten with omega-3 fatty acids, making them beacons of health.

When navigating the waters of seafood selection, We should keep in mind the consequences that reach far beyond our kitchens into the very ecosystems that cradle our blue planet. The call for sustainable choices rings clear: Respect the delicate balance of marine life to ensure the bounty of the seas remains available for generations yet unborn. Line-caught options should be prioritized over net-caught, and we should aim to eat abundant species rather than those that are dwindling. This embraces the interconnection of all life and offers a pledge to tread lightly upon the earth while partaking in its abundance.

Simplicity is the guiding star of seafood preparation. Grilling enhances the natural sweetness of scallops; broiling interweaves salmon's richness with the crisp char of its edges; and baking preserves cod's moist tenderness.

Imagine, if you will, a dish where the succulent and inviting pink curves of shrimp combine with the vibrant hues of bell peppers and the earthy tones of garlic—a stir-fry that speaks of faraway lands and the simple joy of eating well. Or you might prefer a platter of mussels bathed in a broth of white wine and anti-inflammatory herbs like basil and rosemary.

A simple yet profound joy awaits you in seafood chowder, where pieces of firm white fish, potatoes, and corn find harmony in a broth enriched with cream. A seafood paella offers a broad and welcoming canvas with saffron lending its golden hue to the rice—a bed upon which clams, shrimp, and mussels can lay in a resplendent array.

The journey through the preparation of seafood is a path that acknowledges the sea's gifts, accepts them with gratitude, and commits to their preservation.

With seafood, the lightness of fare meets the depth of nourishment, and the table becomes a place of connection—not just with our immediate circle but to the broader world and its ecosystems. Each dish is a culmination of choices made with care, serving not merely to end our hunger but to nourish our bodies and our world on a multitude of levels.

Meaty Meals: Choosing the Right Proteins

Enjoying effective anti-inflammatory meat-based meals involves a nuanced understanding of nutrition, ethics, and taste. The process of selecting animal sources of protein demands not just a keen eye but a depth of knowledge about the provenance and impact of the meats that grace our tables. The need to choose lean meats emerges from a confluence of health considerations and culinary preferences—a balance that seeks to minimize the intake of saturated fats while maximizing the sensory pleasure derived from each bite. This deliberate choice is underscored by an awareness of the heart's needs and the body's inflammatory response to various fats, and by making well-informed decisions, you can elevate the act of meat selection to become a cornerstone of responsible eating.

As we consider the ethical implications of our choices alongside their health impacts, the preference for grass-fed and organic options becomes a testament to a holistic view of health that encompasses not only us, as individuals, but the environment at large. Grass-fed meats are nurtured on a diet that echoes their natural inclinations, and they offer a nutritional profile rich in omega-3 fatty acids and antioxidants. Organic meats are raised without synthetic interventions, meaning that they not only speak to a commitment to purity and sustainability but also are free from any inflammation-prompting pesticides or fertilizers. This dual commitment to grass-fed and organic options, while at times challenging to fulfill, stands as an ideal toward which our dietary practices should aspire.

Marinades and rubs provide avenues for enhancing the flavor of our meat-based meals without resorting to the addition of excessive calories or inflammatory agents. The acids and herbs of marinades tenderize and imbue the meat with depth. Olive oil—with its monounsaturated fats and polyphenols—can be combined with the brightness of lemon and the warmth of garlic, for instance. Rubs involve spices that are ground to release their essential oils, and they can be used to coat the surface of meats, thus creating a crust that seals in juices and introduces a complexity of taste. This exploration of flavors should be guided by an understanding of the healthful properties of various herbs and spices to elevate the preparation of meaty meals to an art form where nutrition and pleasure find their perfect balance.

Accompanying these carefully chosen and seasoned proteins, an array of vegetables and whole grains stands ready to complete the meal. The inclusion of these accompaniments plays a crucial role in the architecture of the meal, ensuring a balance not just of flavors but of nutrients. Vegetables complement the proteins and ensure that you are getting a broad spectrum of vitamins and minerals. Whole grains sustain satiety and provide a counterpoint to the richness of the meats. This harmony of components underscores the principles of anti-inflammatory eating where diversity and balance reign supreme, and each meal becomes an opportunity to nurture the body in its entirety.

As the day yields to the embrace of night and the kitchen becomes a place of gathering and gratitude, the preparation of anti-inflammatory dinners transcends the mundane, subsequently becoming a celebration of nourishment and togetherness. The choices you make can reflect a deep understanding of the interconnectedness of health, taste, and environmental stewardship. This approach will transform the act of eating into an expression of care, for yourself and for the planet.

In this exploration, we have found not just dinner ideas but also principles for living that resonate with our deepest values. As we move forward, let's carry with us the lessons gleaned from this chapter—a commitment to thoughtful ingredient selection, preparation, and pairing that honors the complexity of our needs, the dietary impacts on our inflammation levels, and the richness of the world we inhabit.

Chapter 7:

Twilight Temptations—Offering Snacks With Anti-Inflammatory Intent

So many of us crave a sweet or salty treat after dinner. As our energy levels lag and boredom sets in, our dopamine receptors crave some instant gratification in the form of sweetness and our blood pressure often longs for the boost of some salt intake. But in the context of an anti-inflammatory diet, the crafting of our late-night snacks takes on a new dimension—a fusion of indulgence and mindfulness, where every ingredient is chosen not just for its flavor but for its capacity to nourish and heal. This chapter discusses the ways in which we can ensure that sweetness meets wellness and savory snacks avoid prompting swelling, exploring the delicate balance between treating the palate and nurturing the body.

Sweet Treats With Anti-Inflammatory Benefits

Natural Sweeteners: A Spoonful of Nature's Best

In the pursuit of sweetness, the natural world offers a bounty of options that can enhance flavors without the need for refined sugars. Honey drips with the essence of floral nectars and antimicrobial and antioxidant properties—a testament to its role as a healer throughout history. Maple syrup, with its deep amber hue, carries not just sweetness but a suite of minerals, like manganese and zinc, that are essential for immune system health. Dates are nature's candy, offering a dense sweetness while providing fiber, vitamins, and minerals. Integrating these natural sweeteners into your desserts transforms the act of indulgence into one of kindness toward your body.

Fruit-Based Desserts: The Sweetness of Simplicity

The simple act of baking apples, their cores filled with nuts and spices, fills the air with a fragrance that speaks of comfort and nostalgia. Fruit-based desserts—whether it's a vibrant berry crumble on a warm evening or a refreshing fruit salad kissed with mint—celebrate natural sweetness while providing a feast of antioxidants, fibers, and vitamins. In their simplicity, these desserts embody the philosophy that food can be both a pleasure and a pillar of health.

Dark Chocolate: Decadence with Benefits

Dark chocolate whispers of forbidden indulgence, yet within its rich depths lies a trove of polyphenols (notably flavonoids) known for their anti-inflammatory and antioxidant prowess. The key, however, lies in selection—choosing dark chocolate with a high percentage of cocoa ensures maximum benefits with minimal added sugars. Use it to complement fruits or create dense, satisfying morsels that speak of indulgence without regret. Allowing dark chocolate to play a starring role in your desserts marries the sensory delight of sweetness with the underlying promise of health.

Recipe Ideas: Creativity in the Kitchen

Recipes are not just instructions but also inspiration guiding the creation of desserts that delight the senses while nurturing the body. A no-bake tart with a crust made from ground nuts and dates filled with a lush lemon-infused avocado cream shows the versatility of natural ingredients. Likewise, a batch of energy bites containing oats, chia seeds, almond butter, and a touch of honey offers a quick sweet fix packed with nutrients and anti-inflammatory benefits. The understanding that desserts can be both delightful and healthful invites experimentation and adaptation, consequently encouraging a personal journey through the world of sweet indulgence informed by the principles of anti-inflammatory eating.

When sweetness intersects with wellness, the creation of desserts becomes a practice infused with mindfulness and care. Focusing on the natural sources of sweetness above and exploring recipes rich in anti-inflammatory ingredients reflects a broader philosophy that recognizes the complexity of human health and the simple pleasures of taste.

To maintain low levels of inflammation, your approach to dessert should be guided by the knowledge that what you consume can either nurture or negate your well-being. This offers a path that honors your body's needs while satisfying your cravings and preventing any sense of deprivation that could lead to impulse binges of inflammatory junk food.

Savory Snacks: Crunchy, Salty, and Satisfying

The craving for salty snacks is more than a mere whim of appetite, and it calls for a response that combines the satisfaction of crunch and salt with the body's deeper need for nourishment that supports its complex machinery.

Healthy Chips and Crackers: Innovations From Hearth and Earth

The transformation of vegetables and whole grains into chips and crackers turns the base materials of nature into culinary gold. Thinly sliced zucchini seasoned with sea salt and the faint heat of paprika and baked until each piece has a delicate crispness offers an alternative to the store-bought varieties laden with oils and preservatives. I've even found that these make the perfect base for bite-sized "pizzas," and I love topping them with some tomato and basil puree and a dollop of soft goat cheese before popping them in the oven for five minutes. I've even served these for movie nights with my friends—a scenario that's usually laden with chips, candy, and a whole host of inflammatory temptations—and they go down a treat! Similarly, crackers can be made from whole grain flours with seeds like flax and sesame; each batch of these creations is a small act of rebellion against the processed and the artificial.

Nuts and Seeds: The Lore of the Ancients in Each Bite

Within the compact form of nuts and seeds lies a history as old as civilization itself. The modern kitchen breathes new life into these ancient staples with its array of spices and seasonings. Almonds can be tossed with rosemary and a hint of garlic and roasted to deepen their flavor and enhance their crunch. Pumpkin seeds hide the promise of magnesium and zinc in their green shells, and they are extra delicious when dusted with turmeric and a pinch of black pepper to enhance absorption. These convenient bite-sized morsels of goodness offer not just a snack but a path toward healing and inflammation prevention.

Popcorn: A Canvas for Culinary Creativity

Air-popped to avoid the unnecessary addition of oils, popcorn stands ready to receive a dusting of nutritional yeast for a cheesy richness without the dairy, a sprinkle of smoked paprika for depth, or a light coating of a spice blend that sings with the flavors of distant markets and sun-drenched fields. This option is humble in its origins, but it elevates the act of snacking to delight your palate while adhering to the principles of health and well-being.

Dips and Spreads: The Alchemy of the Blender

Your blender can be a tool not just for the smooth and the liquid but for the creation of dips and spreads that transform the raw and the cooked into creamy concoctions of flavor and health. Garbanzo beans can be softened by cooking and enlivened with the tang of lemon, the richness of tahini, and the piquant bite of garlic, blended into a hummus that's at once familiar and revelatory. The ripe flesh of avocados is laden with healthy fats, and it can merge with cilantro, lime, and a hint of jalapeño to become a guacamole that pairs as well with sliced vegetables as it does with homemade chips and crackers. These spreads stand as pillars of a snack time that satisfies the need for density and flavor without straying from the path of health.

In this exploration of savory snacks, we can see that the act of snacking has the capacity to become a practice of culinary creativity and nutritional wisdom, where each choice reflects your commitment to your well-being and is a celebration of taste.

Smoothies and Juices: Your Antioxidant Fix

Though we discussed the morning potential of smoothies way back in Chapter 4, they—along with juices—offer a swift but nutritionally potent snack any time your body seeks rejuvenation. Far from mere beverages, the crafting of such drinks requires an understanding of ingredients that unite hydration with antioxidants and anti-inflammatory compounds. This section explores the nuanced art of creating beverages that serve as both a pleasure to your palate and a boon to your well-being.

Green Smoothies: The Verdant Elixirs

The allure of green smoothies lies in their ability to disguise the earthiness of leafy greens beneath the vibrant sweetness of fruits. Kale and spinach form the backbone of these elixirs, but their bitterness is tempered with the creamy sweetness of bananas or the tart snap of apples. Avocados introduce healthy fats, therefore transforming the smoothie into a creamy, filling repast. To this verdant base, a sprinkle of chia or flax seeds contributes omega-3 fatty acids, enhancing the anti-inflammatory capabilities of the drink even further. When whirled together, this blend offers a dense infusion of nutrients—a drinkable, delectable salad that invigorates your body with every gulp.

Anti-Inflammatory Juices: Liquid Gold

Juicing is the process of extracting the liquid essence from fruits and vegetables, and it concentrates a wealth of nutrients in a form that our bodies can readily assimilate. The key to crafting juices that fight inflammation lies in the careful selection of ingredients. Carrots and beets provide a foundation rich in antioxidants, while the addition of pineapple or berries introduces a tangy sweetness and a further boost of vitamins.

Ginger and turmeric can lend a spicy warmth to your juice, and their compounds act as natural allies in your body's ongoing battle against inflammation. This golden, vibrant, and inviting shows us the healing potential of a beverage that quenches thirst while soothing inflammation.

Protein Smoothies: The New Builders' Brew

In the quest for muscle repair and growth, protein is a crucial nutrient as the builder of tissues and a source of sustained energy. With their adaptable nature, smoothies provide an ideal medium for integrating plant-based proteins into your diet. Hemp, pea, or rice protein powders can dissolve seamlessly into the base of your smoothie, therefore offering a neutral backdrop that allows the flavors of the other ingredients to shine. Almond or peanut butter lend a creamy thickness to the drink, while a handful of oats introduces complex carbohydrates for energy and satiety. The addition of spinach or kale adds not just a touch of green but a complement of amino acids, consequently rounding out the protein profile of the smoothie. This combination of powerful proteins supports the body's repair mechanisms and provides a delicious aid to recovery and strength.

Hydration and Health: The Dual Promise

At the core of these beverages lies their dual promise: to hydrate and to heal. The act of blending or juicing introduces not just nutrients but water—the most fundamental of needs. Hydration is essential for the optimal functioning of every cell, and it is a vehicle for the distribution and use of antioxidants, vitamins, and minerals within our bodies. The inclusion of ingredients that are high in electrolytes—such as coconut water or citrus fruits—enhances the hydration profile of the drinks. This focus on hydration, paired with the deliberate incorporation of anti-inflammatory ingredients, elevates smoothies and juices from mere beverages to tools of wellness and makes each sip a step toward a more vibrant, healthful state of being.

The diversity and adaptability of these drinks offer a path to hydration and health—a way to infuse your diet with a concentrated dose of nature's healing power. By creating these beverages, the act of drinking thus becomes a deliberate gesture of self-care and a means of nourishing your body with intention and joy.

Homemade Energy Bars and Bites

Making your own energy bars and bites is far removed from the clamor of industrial machinery and the impersonal touch of mass production, and it is a haven for those of us who are seeking sustenance that nourishes both body and spirit. As with so much of the anti-inflammatory diet, the creation of no-bake energy bars and bites is a practice of deliberate ingredient selection based on nutritional profile, capacity to satiate, and ability to impart lasting energy.

The architecture of these compact yet nutritiously dense snacks begins with a foundation of oats, nuts, seeds, and dried fruits. Oats provide a sustained release of energy with their complex carbohydrates and fibers. Almonds, walnuts, and chia seeds lend their textures and flavors to the mix by offering bites that crunch and satisfy in equal measure; they are also a source of protein and anti-inflammatory omega-3s. From the tart sweetness of cranberries to the lush richness of dates, dried fruits act as natural sweeteners while their fibers and vitamins elevate the nutritional content.

The consideration of sweeteners in these creations is a dance between the desire for sweetness and the imperative for health. The overindulgence often inspired by concentrated sugars and refined sweeteners should be avoided in favor of the natural sugars of dates, ripe bananas, and applesauce. When blended and incorporated into the bars and bites, these ingredients impart a sweetness that's impact on our blood sugar levels is moderated by the presence of fibers and nutrients, mitigating rapid spikes. The artistry of using these natural sweeteners lies not just in their health benefits but in their ability to complement and enhance the other ingredients.

The panorama of flavors available in the creation of homemade energy bars and bites is as broad as the imagination. The richness of dark chocolate can be melded with the saltiness of peanut butter for a classic combination that evokes the comforts of childhood while adhering to the principles of anti-inflammatory eating. Dried and chopped tropical fruits can be combined with coconut and almonds for a bite that whispers of sun-drenched afternoons. Finely grated citrus zest can be folded into mixes with cranberries and pistachios, thereby creating bars that sparkle with brightness and crunch. I encourage you to experiment with anti-inflammatory ingredients that you already know you enjoy. This exploration of flavor combinations is bounded only by the limits of creativity and the availability of ingredients, so by its nature, it invites a personal journey through taste, preferences, and nutritional needs.

Crafting homemade energy bars and bites requires no more than the mixing of ingredients and the pressing of the resulting blend into pans or rolling it into balls. Yet, within this simplicity lies a profound act of care and a deliberate choice to consume snacks devoid of additives, preservatives, and the myriad inflammatory unknowns of commercial production.

As the day wanes and the need for a quick source of energy arises, these homemade energy bars and bites stand ready. Additionally, they can be tucked into lunchboxes, perched on desks, or nestled in the recesses of backpacks to offer a moment of snacking respite whenever needed. In the act of reaching for a snack made by your own hands, there lies a connection to the food, a knowledge of its origins, and a trust in its capacity to nourish you deeply. This connection underscores the transformative power of homemade snacks crafted with anti-inflammatory intentions and consumed with gratitude.

Fruit-Based Desserts: Nature's Candy

When the temptation of sugary confections leads to a quagmire of guilt and inflammation, fruit-based desserts provide a path to sweet freedom. Their preparation is often devoid of the complexities and time demands of traditional baking, and they invite a return to the basics, where the natural sweetness of fruits shines bright. This approach not only highlights the inherent flavors and textures of fruits but also aligns with the principles of anti-inflammatory diets.

The allure of these desserts lies not just in their healthful profiles but in the endless possibilities for creativity and presentation. Imagine the vibrant spectacle of fruit skewers: pieces of pineapple, melon, and strawberries—rich in enzymes, vitamins, and antioxidants—threaded onto bamboo sticks creating a mosaic of colors and flavors. This simple yet visually appealing dessert is often accompanied by a dip of citrus-infused Greek yogurt, and it offers a playful and interactive eating experience.

Equally captivating is the concept of stuffed fruits. Peaches have soft and yielding flesh that can become vessels for a filling of crushed almonds and mascarpone lightly sweetened with a drizzle of raw honey. The juxtaposition of textures and the conjunction of flavors in such stuffed fruits demonstrate the versatility of nature's produce.

The innovation extends to the creation of fruit "pizza," where slices of watermelon serve as the base for an array of toppings—from kiwi and berries to a scattering of mint and a dressing of balsamic reduction. This reimagined "pizza" is devoid of flour but rich in phytonutrients and hydration, offering a dessert that's both whimsical and nourishing. A nut-based "crust" that blends ground almonds or cashews with dates and coconut oil can also add a dimension of richness and texture to many dessert options.

Toppings for your fruit-based creations can also be chosen with an eye toward enhancing the nutritional profile while elevating the taste experience. Greek yogurt lends a creamy contrast to the natural sugars of the fruits, and chopped nuts introduce a crunch that complements the soft textures of the fruits, adding a layer of complexity to the dessert. A drizzle of honey or a sprinkle of cinnamon not only sweetens the dish but also brings anti-inflammatory and antimicrobial properties to the table.

The rhythm of the seasons can guide your selection of fruits for these desserts, with each turn of the calendar bringing a new cast of characters to the forefront. Spring's first tender and fragrant strawberries herald the return of color and life, and their sweetness is a perfect match for the lightness of yogurt or the richness of dark chocolate. Summer's bounty—from the lushness of peaches and nectarines to the tartness of cherries—offers a palette of flavors and textures as a reflection of the sun's generosity. Autumn brings the earthy sweetness of apples and pears lending their robust flavors to baking and stuffing. Winter's citrus and pomegranates burst with brightness and vitality—a much-needed reminder of life's cyclical nature during the darker months.

This approach to sweetness, grounded in the gifts of nature and enhanced by thoughtful preparation and presentation, offers a counterpoint to the processed and the artificial—a reminder that in the world of desserts, simplicity and purity can indeed be the highest forms of sophistication.

Decadent Chocolates and Sweets for Special Occasions

When our senses seek to be enchanted and our souls yearn for a touch of sweetness, the allure of chocolate and confections stands unrivaled. The selection of dark chocolate is a declaration of our intent to savor pleasure tempered by the wisdom of moderation. High-quality dark chocolate that is rich in cocoa pleasures the palate with complex notes while offering a guiltless embrace of indulgence with its minimal sugar content and abundant antioxidants. When favoring quality over quantity, the act of selecting good-quality dark chocolate ensures that each bite carries the full spectrum of benefits, ranging from mood elevation to inflammation reduction.

The narrative of indulgence, however, unfolds within the boundaries of moderation. Portion control is not about restriction but rather about ensuring that every confection is a treasure to be unraveled slowly with reverence, which actually enhances our enjoyment in the long run. This practice of moderation extends beyond mere quantity to encompass the time and setting, making these indulgences not everyday occurrences but milestones to be celebrated with the solemnity they deserve. The understanding that these sweets are just one small part of a diet that prioritizes health tempers our urge for excess and guides our hands to reach for just enough to satisfy without tipping the scales of balance. We know that we have plenty of anti-inflammatory sweet treat options that can instead be selected when a small quantity of a larger luxury just won't cut it.

You can also use the crafting of homemade chocolates and sweets as a testament to the joy of eating. Recipes come to life as a reflection of personal taste and an homage to the versatility of chocolate and natural sweeteners. The yielding and rich centers of truffles can be infused with essences of orange or mint. Chocolate bark allows for a medley of toppings ranging from the tartness of dried cherries to the crunch of roasted almonds. These homemade creations combine simple ingredients with the magic of our own hands to create symbols of care crafted not just for the pleasure they bring but for the health they nurture.

Special occasions call for the inclusion of such decadent treats, yet always with an eye for the principles that govern an anti-inflammatory lifestyle. A birthday might find its sweet conclusion in a cake where layers of sponge are enlivened with almond flour, sweetened with maple syrup, and enrobed in a ganache of dark chocolate—its richness cut by the freshness of raspberries. A holiday gathering could be graced by a platter of sweets where dates, stuffed with nut butter and coated in chocolate, offer a nod to tradition while steering the palate toward new territories of taste and health. Occasions that are enriched by the presence of sweets that adhere to the tenets of wellness become not just celebrations but also affirmations of a lifestyle that values health as much as happiness.

In this exploration of chocolates and sweets for special occasions, we can see that there are plenty of options for the integration of these delights into celebrations. Each theme above underscores the possibility of indulgence that aligns with the pursuit of health. The understanding that sweets can be approached with mindfulness and creativity can enhance life's special moments without compromising our well-being, and this offers a bridge between the desire for pleasure and the necessity of health.

As we transition to the next chapter, this journey through the world of anti-inflammatory eating continues toward a deeper understanding of how food shapes our health, moments, and memories.

Chapter 8:

Weaving Wellness Into Life's Fabric

Each day offers a new beginning and fresh opportunities to make choices centered around health and wellness. However, the easiest way to make these impactful decisions day in and day out is to embed them into our routines, preventing us from needing to consciously choose each action each day. Among these routines, exercise is a vital thread that should be interwoven into the fabric of our day, its presence as natural and necessary as the air we breathe. This chapter delves into the integration of exercise into our daily lives by exploring how the many forms of movement can be a wellspring of health, vitality, and joy.

Integrating Exercise Into Your Routine

Tailored Exercise Plans

The notion that one size fits all is a myth, especially when it comes to exercise. Picture a Saturday morning farmers' market: Just as each stall presents a unique array of produce catering to different tastes and needs, exercise routines must be tailored to fit our individual fitness levels and preferences. Start with an honest assessment of where you are and where you hope to be. From there, crafting an exercise plan can center around selecting activities that not only challenge your body but also spark joy and interest. This custom approach ensures sustainability, thus transforming exercise from a fleeting endeavor into a consistent, enjoyable part of life.

Anti-Inflammatory Exercise Benefits

The link between regular, moderate exercise and reduced inflammation is well-documented with studies showing how physical activity can lower levels of inflammatory markers in the body (Godman, 2022). Imagine the bloodstream as a highway; exercise acts as a regulatory force ensuring smooth traffic and preventing the jams that can lead to chronic inflammation. By incorporating activities such as brisk walking, cycling, or swimming into your routine, you engage in a direct dialogue with your body and encourage it to enhance its natural anti-inflammatory responses, thereby supporting your overall well-being.

Variety and Enjoyment

Monotony is the antithesis of motivation. To keep the flame of your enthusiasm burning, you should aim to infuse your exercise routine with variety. Why not swap a session of weight lifting for a dance class? Or replace a solitary run with a group hike? Each activity offers its unique benefits and challenges, ensuring your body and mind remain engaged. A friend of mine even uses her exercise routine as an opportunity to nourish her inner child's dream of joining the circus by taking aerial silks classes. I, on the other hand, love to take any opportunity to run around and goof off outside with my dog. Exercise shouldn't feel like a chore. So, feel free to experiment and find what is fun for you. Seasonal changes provide a perfect opportunity to adjust your routine, inviting you to explore the outdoors in summer or try indoor rock climbing in winter. This rotation not only prevents boredom but also encourages a holistic approach to fitness by addressing different aspects of strength, flexibility, and endurance.

Starting Small

The journey to integrating exercise into your daily life begins with a single step, quite literally. Setting outlandish goals is a sure path to disappointment and injury. Instead, start small. If a 30-minute workout seems daunting, break it down into three 10-minute sessions. Find opportunities for incidental exercise:

Take the stairs instead of the elevator, walk or cycle to work if possible, and stand or take brief walks during long periods of sitting. These small adjustments accumulate, thus building a foundation of fitness and a habit upon which more structured exercises can be layered. It's about making exercise an unobtrusive yet constant presence in your life— barely noticeable on its own but essential to the strength and pattern of a holistically anti-inflammatory lifestyle.

Visual Element: Interactive Exercise Planner

An interactive digital planner can assist you in tailoring your exercise plan by offering a tool for mapping out activities, setting realistic goals, and tracking your progress. There are many such planners available online or as apps for your phone, and they allow for customization based on your personal preferences, fitness levels, and schedules. They're not just guides but companions on your journey to wellness, providing reminders, encouragement, and adjustments to your routine as needed.

The integration of exercise into our daily routines is a testament to our commitment to well-being. It requires no monumental effort, no grand declarations. Instead, it asks for small, consistent steps, a willingness to listen to our bodies, and a desire to consistently introduce movement into our lives.

The Importance of Hydration: Tips for Drinking More Water

Hydration and Inflammation: A Delicate Equilibrium

Hydration plays a pivotal role in a plethora of bodily functions, and as a result, its absence can be hugely detrimental. Every cell and tissue thrives in the presence of adequate water—a medium through which nutrients travel and waste departs. Dehydration can skew this balance, leading to an uptick in inflammation markers. This can easily become an insidious cycle where dehydration exacerbates inflammation, which in turn can lead to further dehydration, creating a negative feedback loop that undermines your body's equilibrium. Proper hydration, therefore, supports processes that mitigate inflammation and fortify your body against its encroachments.

Daily Water Intake Recommendations: A Personalized Blueprint

The quest for optimal hydration is not guided by a universal map; rather, it must acknowledge your individual circumstances; your activity level, climate, and even age play pivotal roles in determining your water needs. For those of us who live rather sedentary lives, the axiom of eight glasses a day provides a baseline, yet for the athletes among us, this amount scarcely scratches the surface. The warmer the climate, the more we sweat, hence heightening our need for replenishment. The balance of adequate hydration is a dynamic equation that demands attentiveness to your body's cues; the color of your urine, for instance, is a vivid indicator, while thirst is a belated sign. Aiming for 1 ml of water per calorie consumed offers an excellent starting point that adjusts with any changes in your lifestyle.

Creative Hydration Ideas: An Alchemy of Flavors

Transforming the act of drinking water from a mundane task to a flavorful journey invites not just consistency in hydration but pleasure. The infusion of water with fruits, herbs, or even vegetables increases the appeal of a simple glass. Cucumber slices and mint offer a refreshment that whispers of spa serenity, while berries and basil merge to create a potion that delights with its complexity. The zest and tang of citrus can imbue water with a vibrancy that invigorates. These infusions are easy to prepare and pleasing to the eye, and they serve as visual and gustatory invitations to sip more, thus turning hydration into an act of anticipation rather than obligation.

Tracking and Reminders: The Guardians of Hydration

With how busy our lives tend to be, it's easy to reach lunchtime only to realize that the only liquids we've drunk have been dehydrating caffeine sources. Technology offers a sentinel in this regard as apps can not only track our water intake but remind us to drink. Setting reminders on devices; creating visual cues in the form of water bottles strategically placed in living and workspaces; or even methodically ticking off a checklist ensures that hydration remains at the forefront of your consciousness.

To enhance your hydration, tailor your strategies to your own needs. Remember that drinking water can be a mindful practice that nourishes and replenishes. In this light, each sip becomes an affirmation of health and a simple yet profound act that commits to a continued anti-inflammatory lifestyle.

Stress Reduction Techniques That Work

Stress carries with it the weight of exacerbating inflammation within the body. Acknowledging this insidious nature of chronic stress demonstrates the imperative need for techniques that mitigate its grasp.

Impact of Stress on Inflammation

Stress finds its way into the crevices of our biological processes, igniting the flames of inflammation. Imagine, if you will, that your body is a walled city with defenses against invaders. Stress acts as a siege that weakens the barriers and gives inflammatory agents free rein within your sanctum. This breach does not merely disturb your body's immediate peace, but it also sets the stage for a protracted struggle in which the body's systems are caught in a relentless battle against the tide of inflammation. In recognizing this, we can see the critical need to fortify the gates through stress management.

Practical Stress Reduction Strategies

To combat stress, a variety of tools stand ready to be wielded with precision and care. Effective time management, for instance, ensures that each task is met not with haste but with the deliberate pace of a well-plotted course. The art of saying "no" can be a sword that slices through the clutter of unnecessary obligations, leaving room for breath and life. Deep breathing exercises help calm the tempest of your mind and return your body to peace. It's also important to set realistic expectations, therefore fostering a harmony between ambition and capability.

Relaxation Techniques

Relaxation techniques provide tranquility amidst the tumult of life. Progressive muscle relaxation, for instance, is a methodical tension and release of each muscle group, and it teaches the body how to step away from a fight-or-flight nervous system response into a rest-and-digest one. Guided imagery allows the mind to voyage to serene landscapes, whether real or conjured, offering a respite from the confines of stress. Aromatherapy involves the ancient dialogue between scent and emotion, utilizing the essence of plants to soothe the mind: Lavender whispers of calm, and peppermint clears the fog of fatigue with each inhalation, for instance.

The Importance of Regular Practice

In the cultivation of a garden, the key to growth lies in the steady nourishment of rain. Similarly, the mitigation of stress through the techniques outlined above demands regularity; the more often you practice these methods during times of calm, the easier and more effective their implementation will be when you're in crisis. This is an iterative process that involves finding the combination of techniques that resonate with you.

As stress and inflammation are so intertwined, the deployment of techniques to untangle this knot is not just an act of healing but an affirmation of your right to a fulfilling life free from inflammatory issues. Amid the ebbs and flows of existence, the capacity to find calm remains within our grasp. From the pragmatic to the meditative, stress management techniques offer a guide to finding peace in the midst of life's storms.

Sleep Hygiene: Restorative Sleep for Healing

Sleep has restorative power and acts as a silent healer within our bodies. This nightly pilgrimage from consciousness to the depths of slumber is more than a mere pause; it's a fundamental ritual in our bodies' ceaseless quest for balance and renewal. As a result, sleep and inflammation have a deeply connected relationship wherein the quality of your rest directly influences your body's inflammatory responses, making sleep an active ally in the pursuit of health.

The Connection Between Sleep and Inflammation

Night is the backdrop against which the body's inflammatory markers are recalibrated. Research illuminates the path sleep takes in moderating these markers by revealing how disruptions in the sleep cycle can lead to an uptick in inflammation and set the stage for a host of chronic conditions to take root (Furman et al., 2022). In contrast, a night of uninterrupted sleep acts as a balm, soothing the fires of inflammation and guiding the body back to a state of equilibrium. It's within this nocturnal sanctuary that damaged cells are repaired, toxins flushed, and the immune system fortified.

Establishing a Sleep Routine

The rhythm of sleep, much like the ebb and flow of tides, thrives on consistency. Cultivating an effective sleep routine is akin to planting a garden; from the pruning of screen time in the hours before bed to the development of a tranquil sleeping environment, each action contributes to the growth of healthy sleep patterns. Dimming lights to mimic the setting sun, choosing bedding that invites relaxation, and maintaining a temperature that whispers of cool breezes also encourage the body to descend into sleep with ease.

Managing Sleep Disturbances

For many, the journey into night is fraught with obstacles, from a restless mind that churns with the day's worries to the body's stubborn refusal to yield to rest. Stress-related insomnia and sleep apnea demand not just acknowledgment but action. Adjustments to your daytime lifestyle can serve as first steps in reclaiming the night; for instance, I now avoid coffee after 3 p.m. and ensure that I get at least 20 minutes of exercise a day to help prep my body for restful slumber.

For those instances where sleep disturbances are ongoing or debilitating, seeking professional guidance can help you understand and overcome these challenges.

Sleep-Aid Practices

Practices that usher in relaxation can be powerful allies in the quest for restful sleep. Mindfulness meditation (discussed below) clears the mind of any clutter of thoughts, and gentle yoga can be used to release the tensions held in your body's memory, thus easing the transition into sleep. When embraced in the quiet of the evening, these practices act as keys that unlock the gates to restorative slumber and guide your body and mind along the healing and rejuvenating path to sleep.

The practices of sleep hygiene are not chore-like tasks but rather gifts we offer ourselves to promote a vital aspect of our bodies' anti-inflammatory processes.

Mindfulness and Meditation: Mental Health Matters

Mindfulness and meditation are ancient yet timeless practices that offer a sanctuary from the relentless pace of life—a haven wherein the mind is invited to shed its burdens and bask in the tranquility of the present moment. Here, in the stillness that these practices cultivate, lies a potent antidote to the inflammation wrought by stress—a gentle recalibration of the body's responses to the external world.

The Benefits of Mindfulness for Inflammation

Mindfulness can guide both your mind and your body toward a state of serene balance. Scientific inquiry peering into the depths of this practice has revealed its capacity to dampen the fires of stress-induced inflammation (Godman, 2022). It acts as a balm, calming the stormy seas within your cellular landscape and reducing your body's production of cytokines. Moreover, the embrace of mindfulness enhances mental resilience and fosters a sense of peace that blankets the psyche with the gentle assurance of well-being.

Getting Started With Meditation

The world of meditation might seem as vast and impenetrable as a dense forest with secrets veiled by the undergrowth of misconceptions and doubts. Yet, the entry into this realm requires no Herculean effort, no leap of faith; rather, it begins with the simplest act of drawing breath. Guided meditations that focus on deep breathing lead the mind through the labyrinth of its own thoughts toward a clearing of calm. To begin engaging with this practice, find a quiet corner where distractions are but distant whispers. This will allow you to sink into the depths of contemplation. It's here, in the interplay of guidance and solitude, that the seeds of a meditation practice are sown, nurtured by consistent effort and the patience to witness your mind's wanderings without judgment.

Integrating Mindfulness Into Daily Activities

Our daily lives offer plenty of fertile ground for the integration of mindfulness by transforming mundane tasks into opportunities for the cultivation of presence. Mindful eating, for instance, transforms each meal into a meditation, where the colors, textures, and flavors of food become objects of contemplation, and their appreciation is a conduit to gratitude and satiety. In-motion mindfulness is also possible, with each step during a walk providing an opportunity to connect with the earth and feel the rhythm of your own movement through space. Even amidst the ebb and flow of work, moments of mindfulness can anchor you by turning the act of breathing into an island of calm in the sea of tasks. This fosters a continuous state of awareness and a gentle undercurrent of calm that runs through the day enriching each moment with the depth of conscious presence.

Resources for Deepening Practice

As your journey into mindfulness and meditation unfolds, you can discover paths that were previously obscured, leading to depths of understanding and realms of peace yet to be explored. Many meditation-oriented resources offer insights and methods to enrich your practice, including apps with a plethora of guided sessions with content tailored to many needs and intentions. Books, too, can illuminate the philosophy and techniques of mindfulness. For those who seek the resonance of shared experiences, local classes and retreats offer sanctuaries of learning—spaces where the collective energy of the practice can elevate your individual journey. These resources are diverse in their forms, and they can serve as catalysts for self-growth by inviting you to delve deeper into the wellspring of mindfulness and explore the boundless potential for peace residing within the quietude of the present moment.

Mindfulness and meditation are modes of existence that infuse daily life with a profound sense of peace and presence. The benefits—extending from the quelling of inflammation to the enhancement of mental health—underscore the integral role these practices play in the architecture of well-being.

Building a Supportive Community for Wellness

The essence of community in health transcends the mere exchange of tips or recipes; it embodies the profound interconnectedness that bonds humans on journeys better taken together. This unity—fostered through shared goals and mutual support—creates a sanctuary of encouragement and accountability, where each member's journey is both personal and part of a larger narrative of communal health.

Discovering like-minded people who also want to live a life less inflamed requires seeking them out in places where wellness is the common language spoken. Online platforms have forums dedicated to anti-inflammatory living, and each post provides a path to collective wisdom, with members offering their insights and companionship. Local wellness groups offer havens of connection too; their meetings and activities are a confluence of like-minded individuals seeking solace and strength in numbers. The sweat and strain of exercise in group fitness classes can also forge bonds of camaraderie, as each shared challenge is a step toward a common goal of health and vitality.

The concept of a wellness circle—a constellation of friends or family members orbiting around the common sun of healthy living—emerges as a beacon of support. This circle thrives on the exchange of nourishing recipes, the collective pursuit of physical activity, and the balm of emotional support. Here, the victories and setbacks of each member find resonance, thereby creating a rhythm of encouragement and empathy that sustains the entire group's momentum. The act of sharing—whether it's a meal rich in anti-inflammatory ingredients or a walk through nature's healing landscapes—becomes a ritual of connection reinforcing the ties that bind the circle.

Amidst the cultivation of personal and shared wellness practices, the act of volunteering and giving back to the broader community weaves an additional layer of purpose into the fabric of well-being. Whether it involves supporting local health initiatives, participating in community clean-ups, or lending a hand at a food bank, this outreach aligns with the principles of anti-inflammatory living by promoting environments and practices that enhance collective well-being.

In the embrace of community, the journey toward a lifestyle that minimizes inflammation and maximizes health finds its strength in the richness of shared experiences. This communal approach to well-being is anchored in the understanding that health is a collective endeavor, and it offers a blueprint for living that honors the interconnectedness of the world at large.

As we close this chapter, we carry with us the understanding that the pursuit of health—particularly in the context of reducing inflammation—is a multifaceted endeavor that thrives on a holistic approach. This recognition paves the way for the exploration of further dimensions of a lifestyle that embraces anti-inflammatory principles, guiding us toward a future where wellness is not just a personal achievement but a shared treasure.

Conclusion

As we stand at the threshold of this journey's end, I invite you to pause and reflect on the path we've traversed together. From the foundational understanding of inflammation to the holistic embrace of diet and lifestyle changes, our expedition has been one of discovery, learning, and most importantly, transformation. We've delved into the complexities of inflammation, identified the villains and heroes on our plates, and explored the pillars of a life less inflamed.

The essence of our journey is a truth both simple and profound: The power to combat inflammation begins with the choices on our forks. The vibrant spectrum of anti-inflammatory foods—from the omega-3 richness of fatty fish to the phytonutrient wealth of colorful vegetables, the ancient wisdom in our spices and herbs, and the life-sustaining energies of berries, nuts, seeds, legumes, and whole grains—results in a symphony in our bodies, tuning it away from inflammation and toward vitality.

Yet, as we've discovered, the melody of well-being is not composed of diet alone. The harmonious integration of exercise, hydration, stress management, restorative sleep, and mindfulness forms the chorus of our anti-inflammatory lives. Each element is a vital note that contributes to the symphony of health and resonates through every cell in our bodies.

I encourage you not to view this book as the final note in your health symphony but as the opening chord. The journey to an anti-inflammatory lifestyle is an ongoing, dynamic process of learning, adapting, and growing. Each day offers a new opportunity to enrich your understanding and tailor these principles to the unique narrative of your life.

So, I urge you to begin your anti-inflammatory journey today. Start small: Swap a processed snack for a handful of berries, take a moment to breathe deeply amidst the day's rush, or simply choose water over soda. Remember, each small choice is a step toward a larger transformation.

Embrace patience and persistence on this path. The journey to reduced inflammation and enhanced well-being is a journey marked by both challenges and triumphs. Celebrate each step, choice, and day you commit to this new way of living.

I also invite you to share your journey with me. Your challenges, successes, and insights can not only enrich your path but also light the way for others embarking on their journey.

In closing, I extend my deepest gratitude to you. Thank you for your trust, time, and willingness to open your heart and mind to this transformative journey. Together, let's step forward into a future defined not by inflammation but by vitality, well-being, and a life lived to its fullest potential.

Here's to your health, happiness, and journey to a life less inflamed.

References

Balakrishna, R., Bjørnerud, T., Bemanian, M., Aune, D., & Fadnes, L. T. (2022). Consumption of nuts and seeds and health outcomes including cardiovascular disease, diabetes and metabolic disease, cancer, and mortality: An umbrella review. *Advances in Nutrition, 13*(6), 2136–2148. https://doi.org/10.1093/advances/nmac077

Bell, J. (2023, September 30). *Health benefits of turmeric and ginger.* https://www.eatingwell.com/article/7561449/health-benefits-of-turmeric-ginger/

Cotter, L. (2017, April 12). *Grab and go breakfast wraps (3 ways).* Cotter Crunch. https://www.cottercrunch.com/grab-and-go-gluten-free-breakfast-wraps/

Cömert, E. D., Mogol, B. A., & Gökmen, V. (2020). Relationship between color and antioxidant capacity of fruits and vegetables. *Current Research in Food Science, 2,* 1–10. https://doi.org/10.1016/j.crfs.2019.11.001

Evans, D. (2024, March 20). *Twenty high-protein vegetarian lunch recipes.* EatingWell. https://www.eatingwell.com/gallery/8050527/high-protein-vegetarian-lunches-for-summer/

5 anti-inflammatory smoothies (2023, February 16). Clean Eating. https://www.cleaneatingmag.com/clean-eating-recipes/clean-beverage-recipes/5-anti-inflammatory-smoothies/

Fleming, A. (2015, January 20). *Creamy anti-inflammatory salad dressing or sauce recipe.* https://www.godairyfree.org/recipes/creamy-anti-inflammatory-salad-dressing

Fresh vs frozen fruit and vegetables—Which are healthier? (2017, September 14). Healthline. https://www.healthline.com/nutrition/fresh-vs-frozen-fruit-and-vegetables

Furman, D., Campisi, J., Verdin, E., Carrera-Bastos, P., Targ, S., Franceschi, C., Ferrucci, L., Gilroy, D. W., Fasano, A., Miller, G. W., Miller, A. H., Mantovani, A., Weyand, C. M., Barzilai, N., Goronzy, J. J., Rando, T. A., Effros, R. B., Lucia, A., Kleinstreuer, N., & Slavich, G. M. (2019). Chronic inflammation in the etiology of disease across the lifespan. *Nature Medicine,* *25*(12), 1822–1832. https://doi.org/10.1038/s41591-019-0675-0

Godman, H. (2022, March 1). *Top ways to reduce daily stress.* Harvard Health. https://www.health.harvard.edu/staying-healthy/top-ways-to-reduce-daily-stress

Goggins, L. (2022, January 28,). *35 anti-inflammatory dinners you can make in one pot.* EatingWell. https://www.eatingwell.com/gallery/7944336/anti-inflammatory-one-pot-dinner-recipes/

Goggins, L. (2022, May 19). *24 anti-inflammatory snacks for a healthy, delicious afternoon.* EatingWell. https://www.eatingwell.com/gallery/7963958/anti-inflammatory-snack-recipes/

Gunnars, K. (2019, December 4). *Grass-fed vs. grain-fed beef—What's the difference?* Healthline. https://www.healthline.com/nutrition/grass-fed-vs-grain-fed-beef

Harvard Health. (2023, April 15). *Quick-start guide to an anti-inflammation diet.* https://www.health.harvard.edu/staying-healthy/quick-start-guide-to-an-antiinflammation-diet

Harvard T.H. Chan School of Public Health. (2021). *Diet review: Anti-inflammatory diet.* https://www.hsph.harvard.edu/nutritionsource/healthy-weight/diet-reviews/anti-inflammatory-diet/

Johnson, J. (2023, March 13). *What are the benefits of bone broth?* MedicalNewsToday. https://www.medicalnewstoday.com/articles/323903?c=96223 0866162

Katz, D. L., Doughty, K., & Ali, A. (2011). Cocoa and chocolate in human health and disease. *Antioxidants & Redox Signaling, 15*(10), 2779. https://doi.org/10.1089/ARS.2010.3697

Klein, L., & Parks, K. (2020). Home meal preparation: A powerful medical intervention. *American Journal of Lifestyle Medicine, 14*(3), 282–285. https://doi.org/10.1177/1559827620907344

LaPlace, L. (2020, July 29) *Fight inflammation by staying hydrated.* Goodwin Living. https://goodwinliving.org/blog/fight-inflammation-by-staying-hydrated/

LeWine, E. H. (2024, March 26). *Foods that fight inflammation.* Harvard Health https://www.health.harvard.edu/staying-healthy/foods-that-fight-inflammation

Nardo, K. (2023, August 31). *High protein waffles (33 grams of protein!).* Eat the Gains. https://eatthegains.com/protein-waffles/

National Institutes of Health. (2023, February 15). *Omega-3 fatty acids fact sheet for health professionals.* Office of Dietary Supplements. https://ods.od.nih.gov/factsheets/Omega3FattyAcids-HealthProfessional/#disc

Raman, R. (2024, February 20). *9 herbs and spices that fight inflammation.* Healthline. https://www.healthline.com/nutrition/anti-inflammatory-herbs

Smith, C. (2021, March 31). *Amazing benefits of overnight oats, according to science.* Eat This Not That. https://www.eatthis.com/benefits-overnight-oats/

Southwick, C. (2023, November 24). *The 7 best anti-inflammatory ingredients to add to your salad.* EatingWell. https://www.eatingwell.com/best-anti-inflammatory-ingredients-for-salads-8406263

U.S. Food & Drug Administration. (2024, March 5). *How to understand and use the nutrition facts label.* https://www.fda.gov/food/nutrition-facts-label/how-understand-and-use-nutrition-facts-label